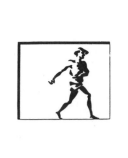

THE BODY CLOCK
DIET BOOK

The Newest Way to
Fast and Permanent
Weight Loss

Ronald Gatty, Ph.D.

SIMON AND SCHUSTER · NEW YORK

DESIGNED BY EVE METZ
MANUFACTURED IN THE UNITED STATES OF AMERICA

1   2   3   4   5   6   7   8   9   10

LIBRARY OF CONGRESS CATALOGING IN PUBLICATION DATA

GATTY, RONALD.
    THE BODY CLOCK DIET BOOK.

    BIBLIOGRAPHY: P.
    INCLUDES INDEX.
    1. REDUCING DIETS.   2. CIRCADIAN RHYTHMS.   I. TITLE.
RM222.2.G39   613.2'5   78-5870
ISBN   0–671–22897–8

The author wishes to thank Simon & Schuster for permission to reprint
the recipe on page 143 from *A Year of Beauty and Health* by Beverly
and Vidal Sassoon, published by Simon and Schuster, copyright ©
1976 by Vidal Sassoon of New York, Inc., and Beverly Sassoon.

ACKNOWLEDGMENTS

This book is dedicated to my students at Baruch College of the City University of New York; in particular, to my former graduate students Drs. Motoki Shirasuka and Joseph X. Nampiaparampil.

Friends and colleagues have been helpful and encouraging, including Drs. Howard R. Moskowitz and Dean Thompson. My brother Alan J. Gatty and Judith Mack have also been of considerable help in preparing the book for publication. Any errors are, of course, my own responsibility, but credit for the new discoveries belongs to all who served on the various research teams. Special credit is due to R. Curtis Graeber, Franz Halberg, Howard Levine, D. D. Makdani, Olaf Mickelsen, and Gordon Williams, in alphabetical order.

RONALD GATTY

CONTENTS

CONTENTS

Part Five: LIVING WITH A WEIGHT-CONTROL PLAN

Part One

YOU ARE WHEN YOU EAT!

1

YOU ARE WHEN YOU EAT—
A WHOLE NEW APPROACH
TO LOSING WEIGHT

This book is written for the average person who is overweight. It is intended to help people to control their weight, to lead healthier lives, to feel better, and to feel better about themselves. To the sound ideas of good nutrition, and those of past diet research, I have added the latest discoveries which really bring weight-loss dieting within reach of almost anyone who wants to lose some poundage.

We have all heard it said so many times: you are what you eat. There is truth to the old saying, although, for most of us, it has not done much to change our behavior. But if you do not eat right, you cannot feel right. Not for long, anyway.

In general, if you eat too many calories you will get fat. Eat foods that lack the necessary nutrients and you will suffer from malnutrition. What we have realized recently, however, is that you are also *when* you eat. This puts a really fresh perspective on natural and proper eating and weight control.

The secret that has eluded science for so long is hidden in the matter of timing. *When you eat during the day can be almost twice as important as the total number of calories you eat.* It is almost twice as important when it comes to that vital matter of accumulating fat—and the buildup or breakdown of the body's solid flesh and muscle. The underlying scientific fact is that both body-

11

weight changes and appetite may be influenced by the timing of food consumption. Calories are less "efficient" in the morning than they are at night—less efficient in adding to body weight. And curiously enough, when we have taken in a lot of our daily food energy early in the day, we don't get so hungry at night. Later I will talk about how we proved that, and I will describe some of the research that brought the new discovery to light.

From this new knowledge, combined with previous nutritional studies, I have developed a pragmatic and nutritionally sound approach to weight-loss dieting. In this book you will learn about the practical implications which apply to your own life. You will see how to integrate this new concept into a lifestyle with a systematic program of good eating and good, healthy living.

In this new approach to weight control we still need balanced meals, the right combination of vitamins and minerals, and the right kind and amount of exercise. What is essentially *new* is that we take into account the natural body rhythms.

A calorie is always a calorie: a measure for the amount of food energy we consume. As a unit of measurement, it is unchangeable. What varies during the different hours of the day is how our body disposes of the food energy we consume. For the moment, consider the body to be like an automobile engine. In a start-up, when the engine is cold, gasoline will be used differently, with different efficiency, than when the engine is warm and running smoothly. The human body needs enough fuel to get started efficiently in the morning and to operate well during the day. But any excess in the evening is likely to be stored as fat. This leads us to some practical advice that runs counter to our usual meal-eating habits.

Most important, any heavy evening meals should be avoided. While most people eat over 70 percent of their daily calories at the evening meal, I suggest that 70 percent of the calories should be eaten at earlier meals, as early as practicable.

In our experiments, people felt less tempted to eat when their heavy meal was in the morning. Also, those calories eaten in the morning quite simply did not add to the body's fat. The main point is summed up by Dr. R. C. Graeber, who coordinated the research project and is now at the Department of Medical Psychophysiology at the Walter Reed Medical Center. In a letter to the Editor of *Ladies' Home Journal*, he wrote, "We did find that mealtiming can affect the amount of body weight gained or lost from the caloric content of food. More specifically, it appears that less weight is gained per calorie when food is consumed in the morning than when it is consumed in the evening. It should be noted that these findings are based on both male and female subjects, none of whom were greatly overweight at the start."

The earliest mention of our scientific breakthrough appeared in a progress report on the research: "From the completed work, pending substantiation on a larger scale, another major and exciting finding emerges, namely that of a relative body weight loss on breakfast. Indeed, there is a relative loss in body weight while subjects eat all they wish for three weeks each day as breakfast only—as compared to three weeks on dinner only, each day."

It is still important, in the case of most overweight people, to reduce the amount of food eaten each day. Virtually all of us overeat to some extent, but now there are ways of making it easier to stop, not only by eating earlier in the day, but also by eating more dietary fiber.

In some quite separate diet experiments, which I helped to design and analyze, we found that bread can be very useful in a weight-reduction program. It helps reduce feelings of hunger so that you feel that you have had enough to eat. There is none of the dizziness or nausea that is associated with low-carbohydrate diets. If the bread contains high levels of fiber, there is even greater weight loss, as well as the added health benefits, now widely recognized, of adding fiber to the diet. The *National Enquirer* carried banner headlines of one of my research reports, claiming that THE MORE BREAD YOU EAT, THE MORE WEIGHT YOU LOSE. That was true of the overweight people in one of our experiments, when high-fiber bread was used. But the people were trying to lose weight in other ways, by cutting down on calories, and especially calorie-rich foods.

What the Body Clock Diet Will Do For You

The Body Clock Diet will do what you have always wanted a diet to do. And there is scientific proof of the new discoveries on which it is based. I have combined these new concepts within the context of the tested, more traditional approaches to weight loss with sound nutrition. The crux of the matter is to eat breakfast like a king, eat lunch like a prince, and eat dinner like a pauper. Your eating should be limited and planned carefully, and you should have a program of regular exercise. Enough knowledge and actual case histories have also been built up to adapt the new discoveries into a practical plan that can be used by just about anyone who wants to become trim and healthy—and to stay that way.

Listen to some typical remarks of people who have tried it.

"I don't know how it happened, really. I noticed the change right away. It was just like you said. I just lost weight! All it seemed to take was shifting much of my day's eating to earlier hours in the day, and making sure I got enough natural fiber. Of course, I deliberately ate less, but it was so easy! I eat less because I don't get hungry later in the day when I start off with a hearty breakfast or brunch. My weight is under control now!" This is how Lynn M. told of losing 18 pounds in two months. She hadn't even increased her exercising much at that time, but she knows that exercise is important, as well as balanced nutrition, regular use of dietary fiber, and early eating of the day's caloric intake.

It is all part of a total program for better health and weight control. Lynn now plans to give up crowded subways and busses to get to work and settle into a routine of brisk walking for at least an hour each day. With that bonus, she will feel better, have better body tone, eventually lower her pulse and heartbeat, and even be able to indulge her whim for an occasional chocolate sundae. She is well on her way to a new life as a curvaceously slender 32-year-old, an attractive wife and a proud mother. She says that her husband takes a lot more interest in her since she has brought her weight under control.

Peter T. also tried the Body Clock Diet. He is an installer for the phone company, a family man, and he is going to night school. Chubby and under a lot of pressure, he told me that nothing had worked to keep him at the weight he wanted to be. He tried fighting the battle of the bulge with various crash diets. He would lose some weight and then find himself right back where he started, overweight and helplessly in front of the refrigerator at 11 P.M., gorging on a Dagwood sandwich. "But when I got into the Body Clock Diet, the pounds seemed to disappear. I didn't seem to feel the need for late-night gorging— once I got used to eating better early in the day. Maybe the high-fiber bread helped too, because I love bread and sandwiches. I just didn't feel so hungry anymore the way I used to. I enjoy my food, but I don't overeat.

"I used to take just a cup of coffee in the morning and run off to work. I didn't feel like eating until midmorning or even noon. Then I'd fill up on coffee-shop stuff—Danish and sugared coffee if it was a snack; hamburger, French fries, and pie if it was a lunch. And boy, I could put away a couple of hamburgers at least. Now I eat more sensibly—but most important, when I got used to shifting my eating up early in the day, I didn't get those cravings later—or at least not so much, anyway. I ate a lot less in the evening and enjoyed it a lot more. I got so I wasn't using food as a way of relieving my tensions. Life seemed to get under control. I even think I began to feel less tense.

"It did take some effort at first to change my old patterns of eating, but somehow, it became easy after a while. It's a diet program I can live with, even like. It seems so natural, and I feel really healthy now. There's no comparison. I'm in control. It's a whole new life! I even joined the Y to get more exercise, and I enjoy it. I used to hate exercise. Even that feels good. Used to be a real drag. I never used to walk when I could ride, even to go to the corner store. Now, I move about a lot on my job, but I still feel the need for a workout on the basketball court once or twice a week. It all feels so natural, and I feel like a new man. I have confidence to do other things I wanted to now that I know I can control my own weight."

Peter's present medical checkups show him in top form. He has lost 32 pounds and has changed his life and the way he feels about himself. He is getting his wife to reduce the same way, though she walks briskly instead of playing basketball. Their two children, Peter Jr. and Mary, at first wondered what was going on. By now they are used to the new meal patterns and they are learning sound nutrition, guided by the Body Clock Diet. They are proud of their parents too, and young Peter likes to join his dad on the basketball court.

Peter and Lynn are typical of the many people who have lost weight by following the Body Clock Diet. The key things to remember are: have nutritious, balanced meals, never indulge in the evening, and take in generous amounts of fiber at all meals. Foods that can harm you, or just not do you any good, should be recognized and avoided. Regular exercise is vital. For some people, it is helpful to begin the commitment to a new life-style by a short-term protein-sparing fast (see Chapter 5). You will thus become more sensitive and respectful of your own body rhythms and treat yourself better on the Body Clock Diet.

2

EVERY DAY IS YOUR BIRTHDAY!

Your exact birth date doesn't matter at all.

Scientists now know that some of our most vital rhythms, called circadian rhythms, occur in about twenty-four-hour cycles. There are also more frequent rhythms within the day, called ultradian rhythms. Then there are longer, slower rhythms that have periods of about a week, a month or a year, called infradian rhythms.

The daily, or circadian, rhythms affect our sleeping and waking, our sexual drive and fertility, our reactions to drugs and medicine, our energy level, alertness and mental–physical coordination, our ability to sense tastes, sound and sight, and, most importantly for our purposes here, our energy level, hunger, digestion, and metabolic use of foods.

Dr. John D. Palmer, a professor at the University of Massachusetts, neatly points up the importance of the daily rhythms: "Because of the living clock's relentless activity, we are not the same person from one hour to the next; but at the same time each day, we are much like we were the day before and much like we will be tomorrow."

The timing of each rhythm is affected by the environment. Other important factors are what we eat, when we eat, how and when we exercise or rest, in what direction and how fast and far we travel, and the particular time-clock schedule and calendar of activity that is often dictated by the society. Because the rhythms are synchronized by our activities and environment, the crucial fact is not the day or even the year of our birth. The crucial fact is whether our many rhythms are in phase with each other and the body system is working optimally for good health.

It would be just a little too simple if all we had to do was consider only our day or year of birth. In truth, your exact birthdate does not matter at all, as far as science can determine. Expressing it more positively, we might say that every day is your birthday. The principal rhythms of the body are the rhythms through which we cycle each and every day. For fortune tellers and astrologers, by contrast, it is the day or moment of birth that is given so much importance. That is convenient for doing their figuring. Almost all of us know our own birthday. It is tempting to hope that by checking our horoscope, we could guide our lives, look forward to adventure, be warned against danger, find certainty in life, or at least hope for better things to come. Astrology assumes there to be rhythms in our lives that depend on the particular moment we were born and the positions of celestial bodies. Our relations with others, it is said, are determined, or at least greatly influenced, by the conjuncture of our cycles and theirs, and the predictable movement of celestial bodies. All this has great historical tradition behind it, and certainly impressive civilizations and great leaders have believed and followed such rhythms, whether or not they exist outside man's mind.

Even in such an important civilization as China, people's personalities have been associated with the year of their birth: the Year of the Rat, the Year of the Snake, the Year of the Hare, and so on. Such speculative ideas are quite fascinating, really. I have looked myself up in the Chinese calendar. And certainly, in the popular magazines and newspapers, I have paused over the horoscope to read what the month or day portends for me and for those I love, according to the dictates of the Zodiac. Haven't you done that? Some of us do it and pretend that it is just for fun. Perhaps underneath, we are curious to read what is said about us, for what more interesting subject is there than ourselves? If only we would admit it, we might be pushed to confess that sometimes it would be nice if we could foresee what the future holds, learn when to be on guard and when we may hope for better things to come. Down deep, maybe we need to believe in something. We seem to need certainty, or at least reassurance, when the reality of life does not provide it.

Perhaps somewhere there is evidence of the usefulness or the truth of astrology, or of the Chinese calendar, of personality traits and fate that depend on the exact time of birth and on the movement of celestial bodies. Such matters are beyond my knowledge and competence, for I have never seen those subjects treated as a science.

The exact day or year of one's birth has never been shown scientifically to explain the many measured rhythms of body and mind that we now recognize as vital to appetite, hunger, body chemistry and weight control. In science, the term for these observable, measured rhythms is "biorhythms."

Unfortunately, when one pronounces the word "biorhythms," the general public thinks of all the publicity that has been given to some unfounded, pseudo-scientific theories that we had better consider right now. There is a great difference between the carefully designed research experiments we have conducted on biorhythms and the completely untested idea that your good and bad days come in relation to just three theoretical rhythms that are supposed to commence on your birthdate.

A dozen popular books, booklets and special calculators help you figure from your birthdate when, supposedly, you will have "critical days." That is when all three computed cycles are bottoming out together. You are told to be careful on those critical days because this is when trouble might occur, either in your health or personal life. It is much like an astrological warning that you are vulnerable mainly at those times.

As we will describe it, the really empirical study of biorhythms encompasses a myriad of observable periodic phenomena, documented in the scientific journals and monographs. The popular version of biorhythms, on the other hand, deals with only three hypothetical rhythms, none of which has ever been documented in the professional scientific literature.

The untested theories date back almost three-quarters of a century to Wilhelm Fliess, who is remembered mostly as a friend and protégé of Sigmund Freud. Fliess wrote a book called *The Rhythm of Life: Foundations of an Exact Biology*. Such a title is exciting and promising but the contents are more fantasy, fiction and fable than fact.

Fliess imagined that our body rhythms begin at the day of birth, though it is obvious that the fetus has rhythms of life prior to birth and, in fact, the particular day of birth may partly depend on caesarian section, or on drugs administered by the doctor. Sensibly enough, Fliess did suggest that we each have a male component and a female component. But he then associated maleness with strength, endurance and courage, and femaleness with sensitivity, intuition and love. That seems to me to be treading on very speculative ground. Are men more courageous than women? Or do they have more endurance? Fliess does not define, measure, or prove these things.

It was even more speculative when Fliess suggested that the male component in each one of us has a twenty-three-day cycle and that the female component has a twenty-eight-day cycle. Most extraordinarily also, he implied that these cycles would remain constant no matter what the environmental influences, such as season, travel across time zones, or work and wake patterns of living that may be required by one's job, such as working on a night shift. He also passed over the effects of diet and exercise, which we will later demonstrate to be of crucial importance.

The appeal is a natural one, that anyone can readily foretell the critical days to come merely by looking up a set of numbers, based on one's birthday. It is almost as easy as checking your horoscope in a newspaper, though it has neither the venerable tradition of astrology nor any evidence to support it. A third cycle was later added, a thirty-three-day creativity cycle of mental acumen and power, again computed rigidly from the day of birth. This idea originally came from an Innsbruck teacher in the nineteen-thirties, again without any sound empirical evidence.

Scientists have examined these hypothetical rhythms, mainly by studying the occurrence of accidents. *Science Digest* reports on an interview with Dr. Jerry Driessen, Research Director for the National Safety Council: "There's no question that our various cycles are important," says Dr. Driessen, and he allows that behavioral cycles may be among them. "But," he points out, "the big question is, why should they begin precisely at birth?"

The Workmen's Compensation Board of British Columbia made a study of occupational accidents with more than 13,000 cases. The Board's research statistician Keith Mason is quoted as concluding: "The results indicated that accidents are no more likely to occur during the so-called critical periods than at any other time." Similarly, the U.S. Tactical Air Command studied 59 aviation accidents to see to what extent they occurred on pilots' critical days. They concluded that the hypothetical critical days contributed nothing to the explanation of the accidents. Further such studies have been made, including one that covered 8625 pilot-involved air accidents. Using records from the Army, Navy, National Transportation Safety Board and the Federal Aviation Agency, four flight safety experts concluded again that the hypothetical critical days were in no way a causal factor.

I have myself examined some of the claims made by the popular writers and advertisers who are proponents of the theory of good and bad luck following three rigidly computed cycles. There is apparently no real evidence supporting the case. One would not take them seriously except that the public seems to accept the ideas without substantiation, or is prone to believing the advertising without question. Certainly the ideas have sold a lot of books and calculators. Perhaps there is something in each one of us that wants to believe there is such a crystal ball to the future and a rationale for the past.

The truth is that we *can* discern our own daily, weekly,

monthly, seasonal and annual rhythms if we take the trouble
to be sensitive to them, to let ourselves feel them consciously,
to monitor them and to study ourselves closely. It does require
some patience and interest in our own bodies and minds, and
some self-observation. Certain of the rhythms, if we are interested in verifying the details, do require periodic analysis of
urine or blood samples. But even without taking such measurements, we can generalize from what is known already, measured
in other people who have participated in scientific experiments.
For the most part, these averages will apply to you too. This is the
real science of human Chronobiology: documenting and measuring actual biorhythms observed in people, not just based on
speculation or unfounded theory.

If you have the inclination to look into the three hypothetical
cycles, by all means do so and enjoy it as a game. There are
tables and charts, easily available by mail-order, or plastic slide-
rule type calculators advertised at impressive prices in the popular press and in the back pages of some magazines. The advertisers will suggest that one can predict the outcome of a football
game, the deaths of movie stars, home runs in baseball, and will
even claim to explain the disaster of Custer's last stand against
the Indians. You might assume it is all true because you can
even buy a $29.95 electronic pocket calculator that will compute
the cycles for you with instant ease. All this might be fun even
if it is not true. Just keep those calculations quite separate from
the biological rhythms that pulse through you every minute of
the day and night, and form the basis for the Body Clock Diet.
These are the very real rhythms that we know relate to your own
personal health and your own personal weight changes.

The most important rhythms for people are the ones that go
through a cycle every day and are basic to our biology. We live
mainly in daily rhythmic processes, and for this reason, we might
claim that your exact birthdate doesn't really matter. Every day
is your birthday.

Part Two

YOUR BASIC ATTITUDES AND DECISIONS

3

IT IS NOT YOUR FAULT YOU ARE FAT!

First of all, let us call a thing by its name. You are fat. Say it to yourself. Recognize the fact. Stay aware of it. Keep reminding yourself of it. It will not do any good to let your awareness of it slip away from your conscious mind. No reproaches, just admission of the fact and awareness of it at all times, at this stage of your treatment. It may not be your fault but it is a fact that you are too fat. Have you got a photo of yourself? I mean a really ugly one that embarrasses you? Prop it up where you can see it. Carry it with you. That is the old you and you will want to remember what you were like. The comparison will strike you as funny some day and you will be proud of yourself, being able to look at the before-and-after difference.

Fatness, or a tendency to fatness, is not a sometime thing. Once it has been established, the tendency will always be with you. By having been fat once, you have more fat cells in your body, and the greater number of them have been enlarged to have a greater capacity for storing more fat. Those fat cells are ready and waiting. Until your new life-style is well established, you will have to maintain a constant vigilance, a constant awareness of that excess weight, or your potential for it. We have ways of making it a lot easier for you now, and it starts with self-awareness.

25

YOUR BASIC ATTITUDES AND DECISIONS

You are not about to escape the reality of fatness by avoiding thinking about it. We cannot deal with a problem by ignoring it, by hiding from it. At the beginning, it is during those moments of relapse—and it only takes a few seconds—when we are likely to gorge, to put back some discouraging pounds, to panic and rush back to the security of excessive eating and the old habits associated with it.

Later, when you are your proper weight and you have adapted to the new life-style, the new attitudes and the new behavior, you will be able to afford to forget that once upon a time you were fat. I do not want you to feel guilty about being fat. But, for the time being, I do not want you to let stray far from your mind the idea that in your own eyes, by your own admission, you are fat. I knew one person who used to tie a string around his finger. People would ask him what it was for and he would smile and mumble an answer. They were curious but they really did not care that much. After a while it became more convenient for him to put a pin in his lapel, no matter what coat he was wearing. It was just a private reminder, especially useful during those first weeks. You do not have to broadcast your feelings about yourself to the world, though others also probably think you are fat! Just keep in mind that you have a special problem of weight control, even if it is not your fault.

You feel fat, or you would not be reading this book, unless you are one of those rare people who wants to gain weight and will use these new concepts for that purpose. For most people the problem is that of being overweight.

Should we use the word "obese" instead of "overweight"? There is a difference. Obesity is a condition of excess body *fat* according to generally accepted medical judgment. Overweight is a condition of excess body *weight*, by your own judgment and preference, or according to the normal range of weights in the population, for your height, sex, and age group. "Overweight" is sometimes used as a more polite term for "obesity."

IT IS NOT YOUR FAULT YOU ARE FAT!

You Are Not Alone

Do not feel that you are alone with the problem. The American Medical Association says that one in five people is overweight. Other authorities put the figure at twice that. It is one of the commonest health problems in the United States and Western Europe. Looked at as a medical problem, obesity would be called epidemic if it had appeared suddenly as a problem. Because obesity has been with the Western world for many decades, we are more likely now to say that it is pandemic—that is, it occurs over a wide geographic area and affects a high proportion of the population.

If obesity were a new problem and were attributable to a single cause, say a microbe or the bite of a mosquito, it would be reason for national and even international alarm. For the threat of swine flu, the U. S. Government mobilized the medical profession and health facilities for an all-out campaign, costing a fortune in taxpayers' dollars. But fatness, or obesity, has been with us longer and is not dramatically new or newsworthy. There has been no great publicized drama of finding a "cure."

Obesity is not a single disease with a single cause or a single cure. But it is the result of our body's responding to our eating habits. In some cases, the body is vulnerable to obesity due to genetic inheritance or glandular disturbances. More commonly, given whatever genetic background we have, it is due to over-eating that is the result of learned, social ways of serving food, of eating food and thinking about food. If fault there be, then it is the fault of our society, not your personal fault or mine.

Dr. George V. Mann of the National Heart and Lung Institute tells us, "Only a small proportion of obese patients have an underlying disease that accounts for their excessive weight." It is just as well to get that medical checkup, but most likely your problem is that you were born with a body that is very efficient in making and storing fat. The way you were born is not your fault. And then your super-efficient fat-producing and fat-storing body has been raised in a society that has developed some crazy, mixed-up ideas about food and eating, and vicious preju-

27

dices against the fat people who are the victims society has created.

People who are overweight according to the "normal" ranges in statistical tables may be one of the last minorities against whom society is prejudiced. In its prejudice, society ignores the fact that half of the people have to be above the median average weight because that is the definition of the median average. We have recognized society's prejudice against Blacks, against Latins, and against women. Perhaps it is time we recognized the prejudice against people who are considered overweight. In the United States we have heard the Blacks claim that Black is Beautiful. In New York there is one group of overweight people who say that Fat is Beautiful!

People Are Different

From my own experience living in the South Sea Islands, I can usually tell the difference among Tahitians, Samoans, and Fijians, even at a distance, from their shapes, although their diets are about the same. Tahitians have a higher proportion of people with a slender build, and the larger Tahitians tend to be fat rather than muscular. Among Samoans there are fewer ectomorphs; many of the people are bulky, although with men, the bulk is often quite firm flesh and muscle, rather than fat. Fiji Islanders are often of medium build (mesomorphs) and quite muscular. Physical anthropologists document these racial or geographic differences among peoples and try to classify the various breeds and racial stocks.

What is relevant for our purposes is to appreciate that these differences do exist, and that some of us have a natural proclivity to store fat that is part of our own heredity, not necessarily the result of overeating or of some glandular disturbance. Hottentots happen to store a large amount of fat in their rumps, making their bottoms protrude in a way that seems unusual. Would you blame them for the shape of their bottoms?

It is perfectly obvious to any farmer or person of rural background that some breeds of animal get fatter easier than others. Stock breeders select their breeds of animals with care when they want heavy feeders and fat animals. Australians use one variety of Merino sheep when their main interest is wool production and another variety when their main interest is meat production. For beef production a farmer might select an Aberdeen Angus, for milk production, perhaps a Jersey cow. There may not be so much variety and specialized development among human beings, but there certainly is a great deal.

Until fairly recently this was not appreciated, even by some medical researchers. Slimming clubs in England were receiving complaints from some members that, although they followed the recommended diet closely, they did not lose weight. Doctors were inclined to think that these dieters had cheated, maybe not deliberately or even consciously, but that one way or another they were taking in uncounted calories.

D. S. Miller of Queen Elizabeth College in London studied 29 women who claimed to be unable to lose weight on the Slimming Club's diet of 1000 to 1500 calories per day, although they had been trying for at least six months. He packed them off to an isolated country home, searched their luggage on arrival for any possible smuggled food, and kept them there for three weeks, all with the women's approval, of course. They were allowed freedom of the grounds, but were permitted to go farther only when accompanied by a member of the staff.

The ladies were kept busy with a program of beauty and relaxation treatments, and with lectures and discussions in the evenings. A dietitian planned and supervised each meal, and every portion of food or waste was measured from each plate. No woman ate more than 1500 calories a day, and the average was measured to be 1350.

Every morning the women were weighed at exactly the same time, after getting up and going to the bathroom, but before breakfast. For seven consecutive days during the experiment, the women each kept a minute-by-minute diary of their activities, and scientists computed the energy expenditure of each, as well as the standard activity of bicycle pedaling at 100 r.p.m. Only 19 of the 29 women lost more than a pound during the whole three weeks. Nine of the women just could not lose weight at all on the weight-reducing diet.

It was proven definitively that those women who could not lose weight on that diet program had remarkably low energy requirements. Their metabolism was operating at a very low level, that is, they have a very low basal metabolic rate (BMR). This was closely correlated with the number of fat cells in their bodies. That number is determined early in life and remains relatively stable during your adult years, no matter how much weight you gain or lose. People can be fat due to enlarged, stuffed fat cells, or because they have a large number of fat cells in their bodies, or both. Writing in the prestigious medical journal *Lancet*, Miller concludes that "it is possible to have two people of the same weight and fat content, but one of them has a smaller total number of fat cells and greater resistance to slimming." Certainly it was not their fault they were fat; their fatness was not due to any gluttony on their part.

Two-thirds of the women lost weight in this experiment, although they had claimed that they could not in the previous six months or more. These women were clearly deluding themselves in thinking they had followed low calorie diets on their own. Fact is, though, they might still have lost weight eating their deceptive diet, if only they had known to shift their eating to earlier hours of the day.

Pattie K. is a New Jersey housewife and mother of two lovely and rather plump children. She herself has been through a dozen diets but none seems to work permanently. The trouble was that she kept making little exceptions "just this time" and it was a long while before she could even recognize that she was cheating on herself. The difficulty disappeared when she began eating hearty breakfasts. "I didn't know it could be so easy," she said. "With big breakfasts I don't feel like stealing snacks at the wrong hours. And a moderate amount of exercise curbs my appetite. The

30

temptation has gone. Well, let's say that it's a lot easier to stay in control."

Others who strictly followed their traditional diets and still did not lose weight have overcome the problem when they shifted most of their eating to the early daytime hours. Sally Jane P. was unable to lose weight although she ate as little as 1200 calories a day. Then she shifted her major meals to breakfast and lunch rather than dinner, and began a program of exercise. She has coasted down to a comfortable 120 pounds, a loss of 31 pounds over a period of four months.

The Question of Guilt

Once we are addicted to incorrect eating habits, the food seems to put itself into our mouths when we are not even aware that we are eating. It is the way a smoker reaches for another cigarette, while reading or talking, not at all aware that he is doing so. This is the problem that is properly considered addictive eating, the way a smoker smokes addictively, and the alcoholic drinks addictively.

We will be learning how to deal with the problem of addictive eating. For the moment, I am only asserting that one should not attach moral blame to the fact that one is fat. It can be due to heredity, or it may be a question of glandular dysfunction in rare cases. Even if it is a question of addiction, I do not think that blame and guilt feelings will do much to overcome the problem. Addicts feel remorse, but that does not help in dealing with the problem realistically and effectively. According to Jean Mayer, President of Tufts University, "The old view of medicine, that patients are sick because of their sins, including their lack of self-restraint—a view that has been generally abandoned in the Western world even in the matter of alcoholism—still dominates as far as obesity is concerned. Obesity, almost alone among all the pathological conditions, remains a moral issue." Somehow this view of obesity must be overcome.

So far, we have laid aside the question of glandular dysfunction, only because it is obvious that a person is not responsible for his own physical defects, and should not be blamed for them. Nonetheless, it may be helpful to give at least passing notice to obesity when it is the result of other physical conditions.

Part of the problem here is to distinguish obesity as the cause or the result of other health problems. Today scientists are less inclined than before to see everything in terms of a single cause and effect, but tend rather to see that certain health problems occur together—that is, they are associated with each other —and it is problematic to say that any one factor causes obesity.

Weight Plateaux

A further condition has now become widely known among researchers and some of the better general practitioners. Each one of us seems to have various levels of weight which stay with us quite naturally. If we get slender, it is down to a certain level that maintains itself fairly easily, but going below that may be very difficult or even dangerous. It could possibly lead to a loss of appetite and malnutrition, and carried to the extreme, it could become a condition the doctors call anorexia nervosa. (This is a medical condition in which a person virtually stops eating and, although dangerously undernourished, may still be deluded into thinking he or she is too fat.) If we gain weight, it is again to a plateau that is fairly readily maintained.

In my own case, being exactly six feet tall, I find that a minimum weight with extreme dieting is approximately 155 pounds. Going below that is difficult and, in fact, undesirable. At one time my weight went as high as 205 pounds, but never really broke into a much higher range, no matter how many calories I consumed, it seemed. A more "normal" range is 168–175 pounds, and this has been easy to maintain with the Body Clock Diet. I am trying to point out that each of us has a few weight levels or plateaux that are readily maintained, but which take effort to deviate from until we reach the next plateau. These are a sort of metabolic barrier that the body seems to "prefer."

Professor Jean Mayer, an authority on nutrition and weight-loss dieting, has remarked that the human body seems to produce fat more readily after some weight has been lost, and it produces fat more slowly after the body's "preferred" weight has been reestablished. He suggests that glucose may be more readily taken up by the body when fat loss has occurred.

Thus we see that, while a calorie is always a calorie—a unit of energy measurement—it may be treated differently by the body, depending on what weight level we are at and where our own metabolic barriers are established. It may also be treated differently at different hours of the same day, and differently in response to the composition of our foods and the combination in which we eat them.

If you are overweight, you can take advantage of this recent understanding, but first you have to free yourself of your own self-blame. You will be dealing with your problem of weight control realistically, but IT IS NOT YOUR FAULT THAT YOU ARE FAT!

4

GETTING STARTED: HOW MUCH DO YOU WANT TO WEIGH?

A specific goal is essential to success. It is the only way to measure your progress against the standard you are reaching for. The vague desire to lose weight can so readily slip back to idle wishful thinking, permitting an all-too-easy escape in a moment of weakness, and one more opportunity to hold the line against destructive eating will be lost.

Select your proper weight, the weight at which you would like to see yourself, as you were perhaps at some earlier time, or a weight you have dreamed of. Even if you were chubby as a youngster, there is very likely some specific weight level for which you want to strive.

Let fantasy run to romance. If you were falling in love, what size dress would you like to be wearing? Or for men, how much would you like to be able to take in your belt? What does this amount to in pounds to be lost? You can't change your bone structure, so I am not speaking of unrealistic fantasies, but of the possibility, the very real opportunity, of seeing yourself as you will be once you firmly decide to live that dream, to follow that dream into action.

Give rein to fantasy, for it is the promise of success that will lead you on to fulfill your dream. If you can dream it, you can do it. If at times it seems too difficult to keep your goal firmly in mind, it might help to remember the song "The Impossible Dream" from the musical *Man of La Mancha*, and it may give you just the little bit of extra courage you need to get past those moments of doubt. Keep the dream alive: it will give you all the strength you will need until the new life-style becomes an established way of life for you.

Strange, perhaps, to speak of dreams and fantasy when the innovations of the Body Clock Diet are based on scientific experiments. But in science, too, our progress is realized only by first conceiving of a possibility, an idea that challenges us to follow uncharted paths and explore new thoughts. Science, too, is made up of fantasy before it is supported by fact. Dreams are what keep us primed with motivation, and motivation is the key to accomplishment. Without dreams there is no progress: the more vividly you can envision the friendly fantasy, the stronger your motivation will be.

You must want to be thin, really want it so much that you can imagine it happening. Look at yourself in a long mirror, with your clothes off. Start to hate that fat, hate it enough to do something about it—permanently. Jiggle yourself around and prod in flabby places. Then turn your profile and take stock of that paunch that will melt away when you finally decide that that is not the image you want. Ponder your excess pounds. Melt them away with your eyes. Imagine it otherwise. Pull in your stomach and see what you could be like, what you will be like. See the difference and never let it leave your mind when you reach for food. Decide exactly the number of pounds that you want to lose.

Remember from past years, and perhaps past diets, the lower plateau that you reached, and how it pleased you. We all seem to have certain graded levels of weight at which our bodies settle in and remain for a while, until pushed up or down to the next level.

How to Establish Your Ideal Weight

I have more faith in your own sense of your best body weight and in your own individual plateaux than in any statistical "norms" that apply to the population in general. However, you do need some kind of guideline. There are tables of ideal or desired body weights for each sex, age, and height. An insurance company prepared them some twenty years ago from actuarial data. They are still widely reprinted and used as a reference. Look yourself up in Exhibit 4–1, but recognize that much depends on whether you judge your frame to be small, medium, or large. Fair relative indications are glove size and the relative thickness of the bones of the wrist. A glove size of 6½ would suggest a small frame; a size of 7 or 7½ would be approximately a medium frame. Anything above an 8 is usually large. However, this rule doesn't fit everybody.

Another guide is the handy European rule of thumb related to me by Dr. Hans Kaunitz, Professor at Columbia University College of Physicians and Surgeons. He takes your height in centimeters, subtracts one hundred, and this is your desirable weight in kilograms. (One inch equals 2.54 centimeters, and one kilogram equals 2.2 pounds.) He adds or subtracts ten percent, depending on whether your frame is large or small. Dr. Kaunitz himself, by experience, estimates so close to the right figure that he hardly needs to do any calculations. But research has shown that individual doctors have widely varying opinions as to the relative degree of overweight, depending on how fat they are themselves, or how plump their wives or husbands are.

You can figure that you should ideally still have a waistline no larger than you had in your early twenties. If your waist has expanded more than an inch and a half, you are the victim of creeping obesity unless you are pregnant or have given birth. Actually, there should be a gradual decline in body weight after your late twenties, because of the gradual loss of muscle tissue.

Exhibit 4–1. Desirable weight for adults with indoor clothes but without shoes. For nude women, subtract two to four pounds for clothing; for nude men, five to seven pounds. (Table reprinted by permission of Metropolitan Life Insurance Company.)

HOW MUCH DO YOU WANT TO WEIGH?

DESIRABLE WEIGHTS

Weight in Pounds According to Frame (In Indoor Clothing)

	HEIGHT Feet	Inches	SMALL FRAME	MEDIUM FRAME	LARGE FRAME
Men	5	1	112–120	118–129	126–141
of Ages 25	5	2	115–123	121–133	129–144
and Over	5	3	118–126	124–136	132–148
	5	4	121–129	127–139	135–152
	5	5	124–133	130–143	138–156
	5	6	128–137	134–147	142–161
	5	7	132–141	138–152	147–166
	5	8	136–145	142–156	151–170
	5	9	140–150	146–160	155–174
	5	10	144–154	150–165	159–179
	5	11	148–158	154–170	164–184
	6	0	152–162	158–175	168–189
	6	1	156–167	162–180	173–194
	6	2	160–171	167–185	178–199
	6	3	164–175	172–190	182–204
	HEIGHT Feet	Inches	SMALL FRAME	MEDIUM FRAME	LARGE FRAME
Women	4	8	92– 98	96–107	104–119
of Ages 25	4	9	94–101	98–110	106–122
and Over	4	10	96–104	101–113	109–125
	4	11	99–107	104–116	112–128
	5	0	102–110	107–119	115–131
	5	1	105–113	110–122	118–134
	5	2	108–116	113–126	121–138
	5	3	111–119	116–130	125–142
	5	4	114–123	120–135	129–146
	5	5	118–127	124–139	133–150
	5	6	122–131	128–143	137–154
	5	7	126–135	132–147	141–158
	5	8	130–140	136–151	145–163
	5	9	134–144	140–155	149–168
	5	10	138–148	144–159	153–173

For girls between 19 and 25, subtract 1 pound for each year under 25.

37

YOUR BASIC ATTITUDES AND DECISIONS

You should not replace that flesh with fat. But how to estimate the amount of excess fat on your body?

A very general, very approximate rule is that about 17 percent of your total weight should be fat, perhaps as little as 14 percent for men, and as much as 20 percent for women. Women's more gentle curves are partly due to a thicker layer of fat under the skin. They are literally better padded. Dr. J. H. Wilmore, of the University of Arizona, has worked out the basis for a simple way of figuring a man's excess weight based on his total weight and his waistline at the navel. For a 176-pound man who is 39 inches around the waist, the excess weight amounts to 23.4 pounds. You can figure your own excess this way (see Exhibit 4–2), but ultimately rely on your own judgment and experience. Scientists may refine their estimates, using more complicated measurements and different figures for men and women, for youngsters, and for people of different levels of physical condition or age. For all the fancy mathematics, they are at best very crude estimates when you want to apply them to an individual.

Exhibit 4–2. How to estimate your excess weight (men only).*

You can estimate how much weight you should lose that is excess fat. Figure your desirable weight from your total weight and your waistline at the navel. Here are the calculations for a man now weighing 176 pounds, with a 39-inch waist line. Use this only as a rough guide, and rely mainly on your own judgment and wishes; you may well be different from the general averages.

Lean Weight $= 98.42 + (1.08 \times 176 \text{ lb.}) - (4.15 \times 39'')$
$= 98.42 + 190.08 \qquad - 161.85$
$= 126.65$ pounds

Desirable total weight $= 126.65 \div .83 = 152.6$
Excess weight in fat $= 176 - 152.6 = $ **23.4 pounds to be lost**

Adapted from W. R. Boxx and J. R. Chambless, *Management Review,* March 1976. Here we use 83% as the appropriate amount of lean weight. A higher figure of 86% is sometimes given for men.

*Women are more complicated: an estimating procedure is now being developed by Dr. Jack H. Wilmore of the University of Arizona.

HOW MUCH DO YOU WANT TO WEIGH?

A simple guideline for measuring your proper weight is to pinch the flesh at the back of the arm, halfway between the elbow and the shoulder. For a man, more than a half-inch pinch suggests overweight, while for a woman, a three-quarter-inch pinch is acceptable because women usually have more fat immediately under the skin. Clinicians use calipers in their research to measure the changing level of surface in the body. As Dr. Jean Mayer has said, the patient who looks fat usually is, but the diagnosis can be clinched by pinching.

Other researchers may plunge their volunteers underwater to measure specific gravity as a guide to overweight. A U. S. Navy medical officer, Captain Albert Behnke, Jr., was the first to realize that athletes' weights far exceed the normal weights for their heights, but the added weight is largely in muscle, not in fat.

In other parts of the world, other ideals are the rule. For example, Latin and Middle Eastern peoples generally prefer a degree of plumpness in women which would be considered excessive in the United States or in most of Europe. Fashions, too, may change with the times: the beauties of Rubens' paintings or of Greek statuary may be considered overweight by modern taste. Trends may favor narrow or wide hips, a flat or prominent chest, more flesh to love or a scanty frame where bones and angles, rather than curves, prevail.

Health and longevity speak for a spare frame, but glamour and romance carry more weight than any urging by nutritional science. Ultimately, you should plan to please yourself, to feel better about yourself, so that you alone decide how much weight you want to live with—and how much you want to live without. Setting the goal is the first step.

A Positive Attitude About Yourself

For any diet system to have a permanent effect, there must be a profound change in your perception of food, of your way of life, and of yourself. Without that you will lack the fixity of purpose that augurs well for the stability of long-term results.

YOUR BASIC ATTITUDES AND DECISIONS

The first thing is the power of positive thinking. Don't look at it as a time-worn cliché. And don't think of it as an unqualified positive attitude toward food. I mean positive thinking about yourself. You can succeed. You are going to succeed. And you are going to remain successful. Surrender all doubt, and believe in your capacity for success. Faith does move mountains, and faith does require surrender. It is a strength beyond willpower if you can have faith in yourself and never question, never doubt that you are now on the path to a new life-style in a slender body.

No self-reproaches, no recriminations, no guilt or apologies— no self-blame at all, even for mistakes. If you do go off your diet, don't dwell on your error. It is past, so put it out of your mind. Go back to the diet, and continue your diet as before. Just proceed positively. Think thin, act thin, and soon enough you will be. You write the scenario and you act out the role.

You can help yourself with constant repetition of any verbal encouragement to yourself. Don't laugh at the silliness of it. Don't be self-conscious. The best athletes and the best coaches know the value of repetitious verbal pep talks. You can even give them to yourself. It is not childish: it is wise to recognize the child who needs encouragement and moral support inside each one of us, even if we have to pat ourselves on the back or stir ourselves with words to right action with a positive attitude.

Your perception of yourself, your self-image must reach for new heights to accommodate a slender body. A successfully slender you is a new person, and if that perception is fixed firmly in your mind as the way things are going to be, your eating behavior will accommodate it.

"You don't change the individual by changing his diet, you change his diet by changing him," says Dr. Theodore Van Itallie of Columbia University, chairman of the National Academy of Sciences' Committee on Clinical Nutrition. He is right, of course. It is our attitude toward ourselves and toward food that we have to change, and the diet will follow naturally, even easily.

That means that food is no longer your solace, your escape, your friend and comforter under tension, anxiety, boredom, or the force of habit. It is a potential enemy. The exquisite delight of a sense-tingling taste is but an unconscious reach away from almost autonomic gluttonous gorging. Very profoundly we must accept the reality that the first taste is the best pleasure any food can offer, and that first taste can be a seductively dangerous enticement to keep on seeking more pleasure. It is a promise that food will never fulfill. Only constant vigilance can protect you.

This is not a sometime change of attitude I am talking about. It is a categorical, day-by-day commitment. You must not quit or even ease up on the vigilance when you achieve your ideal weight. Your goal is not to lose so many pounds, but rather to keep them off. In a deeper sense, even that is not the goal you aim for directly, but the result. It is the result of achieving a continued feeling of being more attractive and of being in control of your life. It will show as much in your eyes as in your figure, says Jean Nidetch, who lost 72 pounds and founded Weight-Watchers. "In the eyes of overweight people, there always seems to be a shadow, that look of missing out on life. But in the faces of those who've triumphed over their weight, you can read just what it means to emerge into a new world, for those eyes reflect pride, dignity, and self-esteem."

5

IF YOU CAN'T WAIT FOR GRADUAL RESULTS

"How many pounds can I expect to lose in a week?" is the question asked first of any diet program. It reveals, of course, a natural eagerness for quick results, once one's mind is made up to lose weight.

The question implies, though, that the problem is just to lose weight, when by now we should recognize that the real problem is how to keep it lost. Almost all overweight people have at some time managed to lose weight, and have even lost plenty. They haven't all managed to keep it off, which requires a change in attitude toward eating, toward food, and toward one's own figure.

The best approach for personal health is to lose weight gradually. Even a pound or two per week is satisfactory, for within two months, at that rate, you can have about 15 pounds less to carry around.

Getting a Head Start

Nonetheless, it is encouraging to get off to an impressive start. Some would be discouraged without it, and lose the sustained interest to carry the diet through to success. In that case, as long as the long-term attitudinal change occurs, it can be useful to begin with a fast, and then turn to a restricted-calorie, carefully timed diet that you can live with on a permanent, daily basis. The quickest way to lose weight is to stop eating, and that is not really so difficult to do. I myself have experienced it unintentionally, while sailing among the South Pacific Islands. A sudden storm blew out our mainsail, and under a jury rig, without an engine, our boat arrived in port much later than expected. I had water, but no food for five days, and only the first day or two did I feel a little uncomfortable, probably more from fear than from actual hunger. Fasting is made easier because there are no small decisions to hesitate over, no difficult little choices to be made, to eat this or not to eat that.

Fasting has recently been heralded as a new method of dieting, but, in truth, it has a long history, going back to the earliest times in the Bible, and is described in both the Old and the New Testaments. Christians often fast during the period before Easter. Muslims fast during the daylight hours during the month of Ramadan. And both Buddhists and Hindus ascribe a religious value to fasting. Many non-Western religions place a great deal of emphasis on the various aspects of diet and fasting, and seem to be more in tune not only with what goes into the body, but also with what goes on within the body—the natural body rhythms—than has been the case generally in the West. That is now changing.

Fasting will probably give you a feeling of well-being, perhaps even of giddiness. You will probably have no trouble maintaining your normal daily level of activity, and you may even feel that you have more energy than usual.

What the Doctors Say About Fasting

The idea of using a fast as an introduction to a permanent diet is not new. Four-to-nine-day fasts were favorably described by Dr. Walter Bloom of Piedmont Hospital in Atlanta, Georgia, almost a quarter of a century ago (*Metabolism*, vol. 8). Working with nine patients who were hospitalized but free to walk around, he reported average weight loss at over 2½ pounds per day for both men and women. He noted that "fasting is well tolerated for prolonged periods" and that "after an initial short period, hunger is not a problem to the patient if he has free access to water."

Most importantly for long-term results, Dr. Bloom discovered that after the fast, patients were much more able to adapt to a diet of restricted calories than they had been before. This seems to correspond to the layman's impression that the stomach shrinks during a fast, so that one is later satisfied with less food than before. Improvement in confidence and attitude are at least as important as the actual number of pounds shed, which is largely a loss of water at first.

Bloom summarizes the success of the method this way: "The patients have all commented about the absence of hunger and symptoms. The experience of fasting also impressed the patients with these facts: (1) They could lose weight. (2) Food was definitely the major cause of their obesity. (3) They had not been eating simply because they were hungry. (4) They had ample willpower to go without food. (5) After having gone for a week without any food, a reducing diet gave them ample satisfaction. (6) Uniformly, during the fast, they experienced a sense of well-being. Thus, the process of re-educating the patient as to new eating habits is considerably simplified for both physician and for patient."

Just a year earlier in the same journal, scientists Keckwick and Powan reported remarkable weight-loss results with high fat and protein diets. In effect, a fasting person is on a high fat and protein diet as the body's carbohydrate reserves are depleted in the first few days of fasting.

The results can be astonishing. Men shed about a pound a day during a two-month fast, to lose a total of 70 or 80 pounds; women generally lose just under a pound a day for a total of 60 or 70 pounds, according to Dr. Ernst Drenick, chief of the general medical section at Wadsworth Veterans Administration Hospital in Los Angeles.

By 1970 the Deaconess Hospital, a training hospital in Boston for the Harvard Medical School, developed a fasting program to minimize the surgical risk for obese patients. The new concept they added was to offer the fasting patient only a liquid protein diet, supplemented by vitamins and minerals. In this way, loss of muscle tissue is kept at a minimum, while the excess body fat and water is shed. Whether in liquid or powder, this protein-sparing diet became the basis of fasting diets at medical clinics in several major cities. Beth Israel Hospital in Newark, New Jersey, Mt. Sinai Hospital in Cleveland, Ohio, and Cedars of Lebanon Hospital in Florida have all started outpatient clinics for fasting patients.

The Effects of Fasting

Fasting with the aid of a protein supplement is called a protein-sparing fast. It has the advantage of helping you to lose weight, at first mostly water, than a lot of fat tissue, without the loss of lean muscle.

Normally recommended is liquid protein, obtainable without prescription in pharmacies and health food stores. There is a variety of commercial brands, some of them flavored because one of the common basic ingredients is a rather heavy and un-tasteful protein substance called collagen that has been mostly broken down, or "predigested," into its basic amino acids. Alternatively, some medical clinics use protein preparations based on casein (milk protein), egg albumin, complete amino acid mixtures, or even lean meat.

When collagen is used, five ounces a day (ten tablespoons) will provide adequate protein and about 300 calories of energy. A large person might use seven or eight ounces. Some take it straight, but most people find it a little easier to take mixed with water or calorie-free soda. And it is essential to drink at least ten cups of water or calorie-free beverage a day, preferably even more. Equally important are heavy daily supplements, including potassium, calcium and folic acid. The exact requirements should be determined by a physician who has examined your medical condition, and the fast should only be carried out with regular medical attention. Normally it should not extend for longer than a few months, and then only in cases of extreme overweight and under close medical supervision.

Fasting can also be particularly beneficial in gaining control of certain medical conditions. Besides its use in preparing obese patients for surgery, it has been used in the treatment of overweight people suffering from such medical problems as hypertension, diabetes, and hypoglycemia.

Although there are many advantages to fasting, there are strong cautions as well, even when the diet is supported with protein supplements, vitamins and minerals. Dr. Drenick has commented, "The long-range results of fasting, in our experience, are very poor. And, if left to themselves, I would expect 90 percent of the patients would return to their original weight or worse." That's the old problem: The weight is lost, but it promises to return unless we develop a profoundly different lifestyle in relation to food.

There can be other problems, too. Short-term, there is sometimes a bad taste in the mouth and bad breath throughout the fast, due to acetone generated by the process called ketosis. Body fats, or triglycerides, are broken down into glycerol and fatty acids, and the liver converts the fatty acids to acetone and beta-hydroxybutyric acid, which, with oxygen, provides fuel for the body. You are living off your own fat.

There are some other side effects, but they are usually temporary. You may feel faint, or a little giddy, due to carbohydrate withdrawal. Blood pressure goes down, which may be good or bad, depending on your condition. The first day some feel pain in the gut. Others find they lose a little hair and the skin dries out a bit if the proper amount of protein is not maintained. Either constipation or diarrhea may occur in the beginning, but it will not be severe. Of course, since you are not eating solid food, you will have fewer bowel movements, but this is not harmful.

In rare instances, during a long-term fast, serious problems may occur with sodium and potassium depletion, and when there is inadequate protein supplement, it is possible for there to be some damage to the heart and kidneys. If the patient does not drink enough water, there can be a buildup in uric acid, which can aggravate the kidneys. In extreme cases, this can contribute to the formation of kidney stones, or perhaps gout.

For these reasons, fasting should be supplemented with protein and adequate water, and should be carried out under a physician's care. Remember that the point of the fast is to build initial confidence and set the stage for continued control, as long as the overweight patient does not consider fasting itself to be a cure. It can be no more than a way to get started.

Weight loss through fasting will not help you in the long run; only a change in your life-style, in your attitudes, will do that. You must change your outlook before you can change your body. And that is what this book will teach you to do, provided that you follow the advice carefully. It will not be hard, once you see the changes taking place in you, both in your body and in how you feel about yourself.

6

EXERCISE IS AN ESSENTIAL PART OF THE COMMITMENT

Exercise is an essential part of the commitment to control one's weight, quite as important as limiting the amount of food and controlling the time it is eaten. Diet alone is not the answer unless it is part of a change in life-style that includes frequent, regular, and vigorous exercise.

Helpful, yes, but why essential? The reason is that inactivity is as much a characteristic of obesity as is overeating. The fact is that overweight people sometimes eat less than others, and as Donald W. Thomas and Jean Mayer have pointed out, this "may help to explain the frustration and anger experienced by some overweight persons when their claims of moderation are met with knowing smiles" (*Psychology Today*, Sept. 1973). Thomas and Mayer refer to inactivity as the "unlikely villain": based on their research studies, they conclude that it is "a major cause of creeping obesity."

Fat Can Take You by Surprise
Imagine just one hundred calories a day beyond what the body needs. That is, say, a single glass of beer or a soft drink, or a couple of strips of bacon, or just an ounce of cheese, or maybe an orange or a cup of soup—not much food at any one time. That amount of energy can be expended with a brisk

twenty-minute walk, but over a year it amounts to over ten pounds of fat if you do not work it off with exercise. And in five years, it would show up as fifty pounds of excess weight, a serious case of obesity.

It is hard to say whether people tend to become inactive when they are overweight, but we do know that they tend to become overweight when they become less active. Most people become less active as they grow up, and slow down even more when they reach middle age. At the same time as they are becoming less active, their more mature bodies require fewer calories. The result is an expanding waistline for men and plumper hips and thighs for women. It is an unfortunate cycle, and the best way to break out of it is to eat less, to eat earlier, and to exercise more. There really isn't any other way. We are inescapably boxed into that reality.

Over 50 percent of the employed people in the United States are now white-collar workers in fairly sedentary occupations. Many blue-collar workers also have sit-down jobs or stand-up jobs that may be tiring, but that do not actually require much vigorous activity that can burn off many calories. Inactivity, in fact, is the cause of fatigue. You know that on some days when you loll about at home, not doing much of anything, you feel more tired than if you had been highly active.

Unfortunately, inactivity has another side effect: it leads you to eat more than you would with moderate activity. Moderate activity, it has been proven, cuts appetite. Look at Exhibit 6–1 and see how, in a study done by Dr. Jean Mayer, both body weight and the amount of food eaten were higher for people with sedentary occupations than for those in occupations requiring light to medium activity.

Modern conveniences are also impediments to weight-loss: the automobile, the extension phone, the remote control on the television all add pounds of fat to our bodies. Dr. Mayer has pointed out that the American Telephone and Telegraph Company claims an extension phone saves an average of seventy miles of walking in a year. That amounts to about 5000 calories of energy in a

Exhibit 6–1. People with sedentary occupations eat more and weigh more than people in occupations that require light to medium activity. (Adapted from J. Mayer, *Overweight: Causes, Cost, and Control,* 1968, p. 74.)

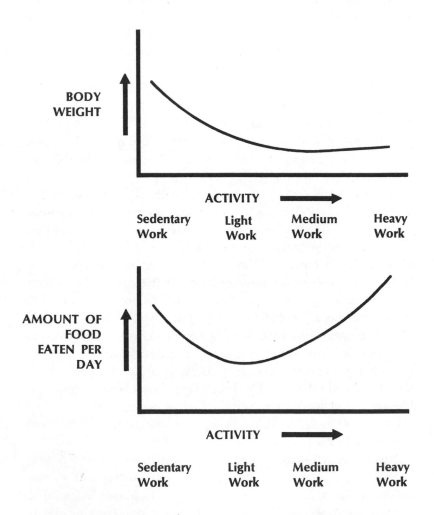

year's time, or about a pound and a half of fat added to your body.

Two Different Kinds of Exercise

There are two aspects to this question of activity and exercise. One is that matter of just burning off energy by keeping active. The second aspect is just as important, I believe, and that is the matter of performing deliberate, regular, vigorous exercises that require sustained and rhythmic intake of air. These are known as aerobic exercises and they include brisk walking, jogging, swimming, and cycling at a conditioning pace. They are exercises that put the heart and lungs to work to maintain a pace and duration that will condition the system for endurance rather than just muscular strength. We owe it to Dr. Kenneth H. Cooper, of the U.S. Air Force Medical Corps, for emphasizing this important distinction in the different types of exercise.

I do not mean to criticize other forms of physical fitness. Muscle-building exercises are fine, as are pushups, situps, or even weight-lifting. And many exercises, such as calisthenics, help with coordination, muscle stretching, and suppleness. Tennis can expend a lot of energy, although it is a stop-start kind that is not usually sustained long enough at a regular pace to qualify as aerobic. Golf provides good fresh air, usually a long and leisurely walk, and momentary bursts of energy while swinging. These are all healthy activities and we should enjoy more of them. But they are not really aerobic exercises. They do not usually leave you out of breath when you are out of condition, although they may tire you and, of course, they burn up calories.

It is not a matter of the activity's being strenuous. Amateur wrestling was my own particular forte as a young man, but the way we trained was as much by running as it was by grunting and groaning with an opponent. Boxers also train more on the road than they do in the ring, and are more likely to be seen at an aerobic exercise like skipping rope than hitting sandbags or a sparring partner.

Out of the arena of sports, and in the household, a person might claim to put in a lot of fatiguing activity just getting Johnny off to school, cleaning house, doing the shopping—always on the run, and certainly tired at the end of the day. It is not the same thing. Those are tiring activities, not conditioning activities. One of the curious facets of aerobic exercises is that they are energizing, not fatiguing. This confounds conventional thinking, but just ask someone who jogs regularly and he will confirm that it gives him a lift to spend a consistent twenty to thirty minutes each day pacing himself to the rhythmic exertion.

Lots of Good Reasons to Exercise

There are lots of good reasons to exercise and it is well to keep them in mind as you begin your own weight-control program:

1. Putting yourself on regular exercise can effect considerable weight loss, not much on any one day, but a great deal over a length of time. My half-hour daily jogging subtracts about ⅔ pound a week. Over the fifty-two weeks of the year, that is a total of 31 pounds! Week by week it is not dramatic, but you could make a mistake and go the other route—gaining 31 pounds a year if each day you ate just one piece of Danish pastry beyond your needs, or forgot the exercises. Do the exercise *and* skip the pastry, and you are ahead of the game by 62 pounds!

You are always expending energy, even when you are asleep, and you might be interested in seeing how many calories are burned up with various activities. The estimates in Exhibit 6–2 are general averages; the actual amounts vary with individuals, depending on their own pace, metabolic rate, and their size. But they give some idea of the relative value of the different activities. Burning off a pound of weight takes about 3500 calories, which is one reason you need some regular, concentrated exercise.

2. Regular, planned exercise is a positive action, something you are doing for yourself. Much of weight control must sound negative, like not eating more than your ration, not eating at all

EXERCISE IS AN ESSENTIAL PART

Exhibit 6–2. Calories expended per minute for various activities. Eight calories is about equivalent to one gram of fat on your body. (Table adapted from L. J. Bogart et al., *Nutrition and Physical Fitness,* 1973, and other sources.)

Activity	Calories per Minute
Sitting, doing nothing	1.5
Sweeping the floor	1.7
Sitting, writing	2
Sitting, playing cards	2.3
Driving a car	2.8
Kneeling, scrubbing	3
Walking, 2½ m.p.h.	3.5
Walking, 3 m.p.h.	4
Ironing clothes	4
Golf	4
Cycling slowly	4–5
Walking, 3½ m.p.h.	5
Gardening, light	5
Waltzing	6
Carpentry	6
Walking, 4½ m.p.h.	7
Tennis	7
Rhumba	7
Gardening, heavy	7
Cycling briskly	7
Horseback riding, trot	8
Calisthenics, vigorous	10
Swimming briskly	10
Squash	10
Skipping rope	10
Jogging	10–13
Running fast	20

in the late night hours. It's a pleasure to find some positive action than can be taken to give you a feeling of being in control, to boost the confidence, the feeling of commitment to be repeated through the week, reminding you frequently that you are getting on top of the problem. Taking such positive, regular action can do wonders for your self-image.

3. Worrisome tension is an enemy of weight control, but tension is worked off by vigorous exercise. Hidden angers or anxieties are pounded out on the pavement or thrashed away in the swimming pool. Worries evaporate with exertion and deep breathing, and the mind clears, freed, some say, to be more creative. A lot of unconscious probes in the refrigerator and snitching of snacks are nothing more than a response to unresolved emotional strains for which vigorous exercise, not food, is the best therapy. Richard Driscoll, staff psychologist at Eastern State Psychiatric Hospital in Knoxville, Tennessee, has reported the favorable effect of jogging on students' nervous anxiety before exams. Other scientists have found similar results.

4. Exercise can moderate the appetite. Adrenaline rises with exercise, and can cut the urge to reach for food; only when you exercise very heavily will the appetite rise to replace much of the energy spent.

5. Although without proof, I am convinced that exercise improves the sexual libido. Both capacity and inclination seem to improve once a conditioning level is reached. Many of us have noticed this but, to my knowledge, no one has yet done a scientific study to prove it. I would be interested in hearing from readers as to how aerobic exercises have affected their sex drives.

More sex means more calories expended, at about 150 calories burned up for each time you make love, according to Dr. Benjamin H. Glover, Associate Professor of Psychology at the University of Wisconsin Medical School in Madison (*Hospital Practice*, June 1977). A healthy sex life can obviously be a big asset to any weight-control program.

6. There are definite improvements in breathing efficiency. A

desk worker normally breathes in about a pint of air, and since his lungs hold six pints of air, we might say that five-sixths of his lungs remains unused. The amount of fresh air reaching your lungs has a lot to do with your energy level: if your breathing is too shallow, you are unwittingly putting yourself on short rations of oxygen! Most people take fourteen to twenty shallow breaths a minute. Normal, healthy conditioning will halve that rate and make for much more efficient, deeper breathing. The vital capacity of the lungs is actually increased as measured by the amount of air you can breathe out from one deep breath. But more: In condition, a person can push as much as twenty times his vital capacity through his lungs in one minute; out of condition, a person might do this only ten times. Muscles of the diaphragm and chest are better developed to get air moved through the system.

7. Your resting heart rate will go down by ten to twenty beats per minute when you maintain yourself in condition. This makes the heart's job easier. Out of condition a resting heart rate of eighty beats per minute might be common; in condition it is more likely to be sixty. At extreme exertion, the conditioned heart peaks at about 190 beats per minute, but out of condition, exertion will cause the heart to pound away at 220 beats per minute.

Generally, it is thought that aerobic exercise improves the size of blood vessels and arteries, allowing better circulation, more volume of blood in the body, more red blood cells, more hemoglobin, and thus more energy. There is some evidence that the heart muscle conditioned by exercise is less prone to cardiac failure. Heart attacks are less likely, according to some medical doctors, although others are waiting for more evidence on that score. Certainly in many cases it lowers the blood pressure: I am a witness to that myself.

8. Further advantages occur in the blood: We have two main kinds of fat in the blood, triglycerides and cholesterol, and both of them may be harmful at high levels, increasing the risk of heart attack. Exercise definitely lowers the triglycerides and in

some cases appears also to lower the serum cholesterol. Actually, serum cholesterol itself may not have all the importance commonly believed. Recent research points to the protein compounds that transport the cholesterol as the actual culprits. These are called lipoproteins ("fat proteins"), and their density seems to be the crucial factor. Low-density carrier proteins carry cholesterol to where it can be accumulated and build up blockages in blood flow. High-density carrier proteins, on the other hand, remove the cholesterol from the arteries and carry it to the liver, where it is broken down and removed as waste. The key, then, it seems, is to keep the low-density proteins at a low level and the high-density proteins at a high level. This is what exercise does.

At the Stanford Heart Disease Prevention Program, Dr. Peter D. Wood and his associates matched a group of middle-aged men who run fifteen miles a week with a group that did no running. Those who did no running had triglyceride levels twice as high and cholesterol levels that were slightly higher. The runners had a high level of lipoprotein, 51 percent above the non-runners, indicating relative immunity from heart attack. Such studies do not definitively prove cause and effect, but the circumstantial evidence is pretty convincing.

9. Perhaps most importantly, being in condition brings on a steady state of physical and mental well-being that many people have never known. It has to be experienced to be understood. It is more than an improved self-image and self-confidence. It amounts to feeling good all over. Thirty-two-year-old Janet S. jogs every weekday around Washington Square in New York City. This morning I asked her to explain how it feels to be in condition. (She has been at it for eight months and during this time has lost eighteen pounds.) She explained, "Well, I know I can do things now. Running every day has changed my life. Now I'm on top of the world. Things don't get to me the way they used to. My head is clear, and I'm more sure of everything I do. I just feel good all the time. And special because it's something I did for myself and by myself. You know how it is because I see you out here every morning jogging, too. You just feel good

all over. You feel right about yourself and the world seems all right, too."

You will sleep better, too. Dr. D. L. F. Dunleavy and his associates have demonstrated that deep sleep (slow-wave sleep) is increased with the increased metabolic rate that exercise brings on (*Hospital Practice*, August 1976, p. 83). Also increased is the flow of growth hormone, important to all of us, but especially to children in their growing years.

10. This may not concern you, if you don't smoke, but there is mounting evidence that aerobic exercise is one of the easiest paths to getting rid of the habit painlessly. It was Dr. Howard R. Moskowitz, President of MPI Sensory Testing, Inc., who first told me that jogging had just replaced his chain smoking as a nervous outlet. "I didn't seem to need the cigarettes anymore. It didn't seem to be important. I'd find the cigarettes sitting around unsmoked. Finally I just threw them out. That was after about six months of daily running." This is worth knowing for the fifty or sixty million Americans who smoke a total of 600 billion cigarettes a year. According to Dr. Gio B. Gori of the National Cancer Institute, tobacco is responsible for 90 percent of the cases of lung cancer, 30 percent of the cases of atherosclerosis (the cause of heart disease), 75 percent of the chronic bronchitis, and 80 percent of the emphysema.

Even as few as ten puffs of a cigarette increase resistance to air that should be reaching the lungs, and the effect lasts for one hour after a smoke. The accumulation of carbon dioxide inhibits as much as 7 percent of the hemoglobin from transporting oxygen.

What happens with sustained jogging is that you find smoking interferes with the exercise, and daily you recognize it as more and more of a nuisance. Everyone I know who has reached physical condition simply lets smoking fall by the wayside, mostly without much difficulty at all. You may find it decreases your drinking of alcohol, too. Alcohol inhibits the release of oxygen from hemoglobin by slowing down the enzymes that affect this. The body just might sense this even if you are not aware of it.

When we are young many of us think that money is the scarce

resource in our lives. Later we may think the number of hours in the day is the limiting resource. It is only in maturity that we finally realize that our own health and vigor is the main limitation in our lives. Like money and time, they are resources that can be conserved only by using them.

This means that we must make time for exercise, especially aerobic exercise. This should be a number-one priority in life, along with controlling the amount and timing of our meals. Nothing is more important.

No Excuses!

You need to devise some kind of regular program for yourself. Thinking over your own situation, though, you may be tempted to excuse yourself for one reason or another. Let's look at some of those reasons carefully and see what merit they have.

1. You have no time. You are too busy. Too busy to look after your own health? Maybe it is sounder thinking to put your health before almost all else. It is the most precious thing you can have and, without it, you are not much help to yourself or to others. The answer is to make time for conditioning exercises.

2. You are leading an active life, on your feet much of the day. You will find conditioning exercise energizing, not tiring. It helps give you endurance for doing other tasks.

3. You're already committed to golf (or tennis, or bowling, et cetera). Good. Now try an aerobic exercise, such as jogging or jumping rope, more often, more regularly. You can hardly get too much regular exercise, and a good part of it should be aerobic.

4. You feel self-conscious—especially if you are overweight— jogging or swimming when others can see you. I know that feeling, but after the first day or two, you get to realize that no one is really staring at you, and it wouldn't make any difference anyway. Now I carry running shoes and old clothes whenever I travel, and in cities around the country, I jog around the neighborhood of the hotel. The hotel doorman gives but a momentary glance. Probably he is thinking that he ought to jog, too. Maybe you need company, others to do it with you. That is not neces-

sary, although it might be more fun if your family and friends join in. Many of us are loners, and would run whether no one else does or everyone else does.

5. You have a medical condition that inhibits your exercise. In very few cases is there any danger, especially if you jog or swim with gentle moderation until you reach condition. Most doctors would be delighted if their patients would get more exercise, as long as they don't push themselves too hard at first. Don't use a medical excuse unless your doctor has given you a checkup recently and expressly advises against getting into condition. Very few would do so.

6. The weather can be a problem and too cozy an excuse not to exercise aerobically. Many of us jog all year round, and the only days we skip are pouring rain, or when there is ice on the pavement. Then we have to go indoors, either at a YMCA, a club, or at home where we can jump rope or jog in place. No problem, really. There aren't any good reasons for not getting in shape, although sometimes we look for excuses. It is time to get cracking and move into action.

People from Every Walk of Life

People from every walk of life have become involved in their own physical condition. Wealth or fame mean nothing if a person is not in good physical shape, and the jogging tracks are filled with prominent people who know they have to get out there and sweat if they want the most from life with good health and a trim figure. Nothing can get you into physical shape except your own efforts. Designer Oleg Cassini regularly jogs two miles around the Gramercy Park area in the heart of Manhattan, right next to Baruch College, City University of New York, where I teach. One of our graduates is Herman Badillo, a prominent New York politician, who at 47 years of age regularly put in twelve miles a week around a baseball lot in Washington, or around his home in the Bronx. Baritone Robert Merrill jogs near his home in the hilly country of Westchester County. He says, "I just listen to my legs and my feet, turn everything off, and my mind becomes very clear." In Central Park you might find Jackie Kennedy Onassis on the run, and along the East River, Shirley MacLaine puts in a fast seven miles, as much as 35 miles some weeks. I see professors and scientists, housewives, and students from both high school and college. If you haven't noticed, it is an egalitarian society that gets out to run and sweat for health and weight control.

How to Go About It

First is breathing. Square your shoulders, blades close to each other, and breathe deeply into the diaphragm. Don't raise or expand the chest. Repeated deep breaths will both relax your tensions and give you energy from the oxygen. Years ago in the South Sea Islands, I used to be a sea-diver for various commercial marine products (trochus shell, bêche-de-mer, some pearl shell), and early on the islanders taught me that slow, full, and deep breathing was just as important on the surface as beneath the sea. It is something we can all learn by practicing each day. Curiously enough, you will find that it revitalizes you, and it also relieves the urge to eat (or smoke) when there is no real underlying hunger.

Second, ignore or bypass a lot of the modern conveniences you have come to depend on. Walk to the post office or the store. Walk briskly to and from work or school. If it is too far to walk all the way, perhaps you could get off the bus a few stops early, or park your car a little farther away from your destination. No matter where you live, you can find ways to increase your opportunities to walk and jog. Many of us are already doing that. My immediate neighbor is a top retail executive in Manhattan, and he walks forty-five blocks each way, each day, and three times a week he does laps around an indoor track at the YMCA. When you have to pick up something from the floor, use the occasion to stretch the muscles gently. Look for opportunities to be active, move about and stretch, using as much effort as possible, especially if the action can exercise the heart and lungs in brisk movement.

EXERCISE IS AN ESSENTIAL PART

You need to work up a sweat in aerobic exercise at least three times a week, and maintain the effort long enough to have a conditioning effect. Normally that would be thirty minutes, certainly no less than twenty. Better still is the regularity of doing it every day, although I think a fair rule is never to let two days pass without aerobic exercise unless there is a severe medical reason urged upon you by your doctor. Regularity and consistency are crucial to maintaining physical condition. Start modestly. Don't dash out, thinking you can suddenly plunge into high levels of performance in the first weeks. It will take three to six months to get your heart and lungs into shape, and your figure will follow. After all, it took years to get out of shape, so you need a few months to get into shape. This means you should begin gradually, even cautiously. When jogging, you might alternate brisk walking with a slow, easy run. Don't strain. Run ploddingly, gently, but run. When you are out of breath, just ease up.

Don't compare yourself with other joggers who are in top condition, breezing by you. There is no competition to win. There is nothing to prove, not even to yourself. Breathe deeply, rhythmically, and feel free to pant. There is nothing wrong with being out of breath as long as you don't strain. It just means that oxygen in your system is temporarily depleted, and lactic acid has been building up in your muscles, the so-called oxygen deficit. Keep walking briskly as you regain your breath. Breathe deeply and freely.

The only equipment that may be helpful is a pair of running shoes, and those only because sidewalks or indoor tracks are hard and the feet take a pounding. You may develop sore muscles or sore feet. That probably means you have been pushing yourself too hard. Ease up but don't give up. A little massaging will help.

We all have different levels of conditioning or deconditioning, so don't bother with comparisons with other people's performances. Suddenly you will notice that it is easy, that your legs run by themselves. You won't be huffing and puffing, you will be just gliding along. Your mind is removed from concentration on the physical exertion. This is what conditioned people sometimes

61

refer to as the Zen of running, which often occurs after the first thirty minutes. You may not experience this for several months. Whether or not you still have some excess weight to lose, within two months or so you will come to enjoy your regular exercise, and to feel that you definitely need and want it.

Figure the Calories You Burn

For the exercise to have the effect of conditioning you, it should sustain your pulse at about 75 percent of your maximum heart rate. Usually that maximum may be figured at 220 minus your age. You can readily count your own pulse at rest, and at the highest level it is raised by your various activities.

A very rough approximation of energy consumption (calories expended per minute) can be figured for any of your activities by counting your own pulse rate when you stop for a minute.

For women: calories/minute = .054 times pulse rate, minus 3.2.

For men: calories/minute = .1 times pulse rate, minus 5.4.

Sustaining your conditioning pulse level for twenty-five minutes or more at high levels will not only burn off calories, it will also have that energizing effect of building up your potential oxygen consumption from the air you breathe.

Getting into condition has a double advantage. Besides feeling better, you will burn off more calories per minute for a given amount of exercise, as measured by your pulse. Even when you are not exercising, you'll be burning off just a little more energy each minute, but the payoff really shows up as you move into action. At a heart rate (pulse) of 120, a person in condition is burning off calories at a rate that is 50 percent higher than he or she would when out of condition.

In or out of physical condition, men seem to have an advantage in burning off more energy for any given level of exertion. (See Exhibit 6–3.) Nonetheless, for a given level of exertion, both men and women benefit by burning off more energy when they are in condition. In other words, they can do more physical work with less effort. That is an advantage in our overfed society. Maybe in ancient times, or among underfed people today, it is

Exhibit 6–3. Training and physical conditioning help both men and women burn off more calories per minute for a given level of exertion as measured by the pulse rate. Men have an advantage over women in burning off more calories more easily, and they benefit slightly more by being physically conditioned through training. (Adapted from P. R. Payne *et al., American Journal of Clinical Nutrition,* September 1971.)

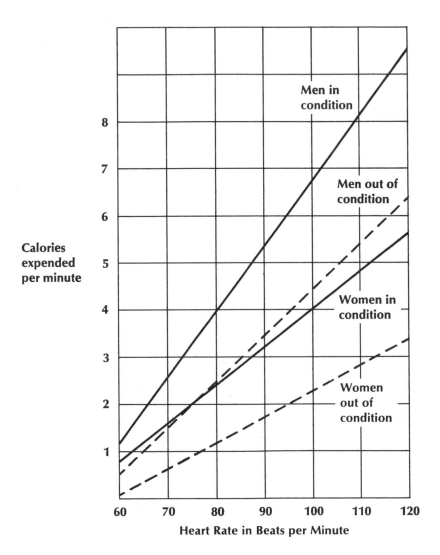

an advantage for human survival that women's bodies conserve energy; in modern times, in our overfed countries, it is no advantage at all.

You may prefer swimming to jogging, or you may like bicycling, skipping rope or cross-country skiing, but there are few activities that can match jogging for simplicity and convenience. At any rate, do not be discouraged by what looks like slow progress at first. Easy does it, and before long you will find the exercise fills a gap in your life that you hardly knew was there. Not only will it help you lose weight, it will give you a feeling of being in control.

Part Three

THE EFFECTS OF
THE BODY CLOCK

7

THESE PEOPLE LOST WEIGHT BY EATING THEIR MEALS EARLIER!

From one hour to the next, our bodies are changing—always in flux, always adapting, always in rhythms. Different internal body processes predominate at different hours, according to the body clock and the body calendar.

We are speaking now of rhythms that affect our digestive processes. This includes the transformation of the calories, or energy in food, to build up and restore the body, provide energy for our physical activities, and to lay by energy in stored form (such as in the body's fat tissues).

When we eat food containing calories, will this be processed differently, or with different efficiency, at different times of the day? And could the timing, as well as the amount and kind of food, affect any weight change of the consumer? The answer is yes to both questions.

The questions are vital from two major points of view. First, in underdeveloped countries where hunger prevails, people might be able to use their limited food to greater advantage by eating their meals at certain hours. Second, in the clinical practice of medicine, it might be possible to administer drugs or other medical treatment timed optimally to the body's rhythms and perhaps even synchronized by the consumption of food.

In this present book we are, of course, more concerned with

timing of meals that would minimize the fattening effect of calories in the overfed countries of the Western World. There are some of us who want our food to be *less* efficient in building up the body's fat.

The First Experiment

A team of researchers at the University of Minnesota Medical School began their work with human diets in 1974, and the first startling results were reported in a paper called, "We are not only what we eat, but when we eat," at the 2nd International Congress on Energy Balance in Man, in Switzerland, in March of that year. These first results were only preliminary, suggestive of the different effects of mealtiming, with data on three people eating a fixed and normal diet of 2000 calories a day.

Later in the same year there were more volunteers for the study, so we may describe it as one experiment with a total of four men and three women. None of them was very overweight or trying to lose weight, but one young lady was a little plump from earlier overeating. The purpose of the experiment was to discern the effect of different mealtimes on body rhythms and on changes in body weight, when the caloric intake was kept at a constant and normal level.

Each person was to endure two weeks on the rigorous experiment. The volunteers agreed to eat only one meal each day, carefully measured, served and eaten at the Clinical Research Center. They would spend one week eating only dinner, at 5:30 P.M., and one week eating only breakfast, at 7 A.M.

Two of the people began with a week of only breakfast each day and the others began with a week of only dinner. After a week, they switched their mealtime to eat at the other time of day, to make this a "crossover" design of experiment. Rations were set at 2000 calories a day for everyone. Food was presented in one of two alternated menus, a breakfast-type menu and a dinner-type menu. The two meals were offered on alternate days, no matter whether the volunteer was restricted to having only breakfast or only dinner. (See Exhibits 7–1 and 7–2.)

Exhibit 7–1. Meal plan for 7 volunteers, eating a fixed 2000 calories/day, alternating each day between a ham & egg meal and a steak & potato meal, and alternating each week between early meals and late meals.

EXPERIMENT BEGINS

Measures of Body Rhythms from blood & urine

Early Meals 2 people	**Late Meals** 5 people
Average weight <u>loss</u> 1.69 lb/week	Average weight <u>gain</u> 1.01 lb/week

One Week

Measures of Body Rhythms from blood & urine

Late Meals	**Early Meals**
Average weight <u>gain</u> .87 lb/week	Average weight <u>loss</u> 1.12 lb/week

One Week

END OF EXPERIMENT

Measures of Body Rhythms from blood & urine

WEIGHT LOSS
Advantage of early meals

2.56 lb/week   2.13 lb/week
Group Average   Group Average

2.34 lb/week
Average of the two Groups

It sounds a little odd to eat breakfast foods at dinner or dinner foods at breakfast, but at least that adds some variety to an otherwise monotonous two weeks. The meals themselves were appetizing and nutritious enough. The breakfast-type menu included fruit juice and tomato juice, two eggs with ham, buttered whole-wheat toast and jelly, breakfast cereal with milk and sugar, raisins and a doughnut. The dinner-type meal included sirloin steak, baked potato, peas and carrots, whole-wheat bread with butter and jelly, orange juice, cherry nectar, applesauce and butterscotch whip for dessert, and a measured amount of sugar.

Each meal totaled very close to 2000 calories, with 250 grams of carbohydrate, 77 grams of protein and 75 grams of fat. Iron was kept at a steady 13 milligrams a day. There is plenty of good nutrition in this daily diet, but to magnify the effect of eating at different hours of the day, the volunteers would eat only that one meal each day. It was difficult for them to resist temptation at other hours, and it would not be sound dietetics to maintain such a meal plan over a long period of time. But those were the demands of the experiment.

Between-meal beverages could also affect body weight, and these were carefully measured and recorded. Only calorie-free beverages were allowed: water, a diet cola, and a sweetened but sugarless lemon drink. The volunteers drank at least 5¼

Exhibit 7–2. "Steak and potato or ham and eggs amount to the same thing." This was a fixed menu of almost 2000 calories/day for the volunteers, with a ham and eggs meal one day and a steak and potato meal the next. The two meals have the same number of calories and basic nutrient content. The diet was designed only for experimental purposes, to test the effect of early versus late meals. It is not intended as a weight-loss diet, or as a recommended diet for the general public. Some foods were included (jelly, sugar, doughnut) just to make the two meals equivalent in nutrients, to add a little variety, and to maintain a level of nutrients and calories that might be typical of a person's normal daily diet. Both meals contain the same amounts of protein (77 g), fat (75 g), and carbohydrate (250 g). Calorie-free beverages were permitted such as coffee, tea, diet soda.

LOSING WEIGHT BY EATING EARLY

HAM & EGGS MEAL

	grams	calories
Tomato juice	120	27
Grape juice	250	165
Cereal	40	158
Raisins	25	72
Sugar	51	204
Milk	360	234
Two eggs	100	179
Ham	120	270
Whole-wheat toast	75	182
Butter	30	221
Jelly	20	57
Doughnut	50	196
Total	1241	1965

STEAK & POTATO MEAL

	grams	calories
Frozen orange juice	240	95
Cherry nectar	130	19
Sirloin steak	200	250
Baked potato	200	152
Frozen peas	100	68
Canned carrots	100	25
Whole-wheat bread	90	219
Butter	55	389
Jelly	20	57
Milk	360	234
Applesauce	200	82
Sugar	41	164
Butterscotch whip	140	207
Total	1876	1961

pints a day. In addition to mealtime beverages, they were to drink a little more than a cupful of liquid every two hours, though they could have more if they wished.

Everyone Lost Weight with Early Meals

Now for the crucial matter of monitoring the volunteers' gain or loss of weight on the morning diet and the evening diet. Each person was weighed at regular intervals, three to five times a day, wearing clothes but no shoes, and just after urinating.

The result was that everyone lost weight when the meal was eaten early in the day and all except one person gained weight when the meal was eaten late in the day.

Average weight loss of individuals on early meals was about 1.28 pounds in the week, while weight gain with late meals averaged .97 pound. The difference between a 1.28 pound loss (early meals) and a .97 pound gain (late meals) is the net advantage of early meals, close to 2.25 pounds in just one week. Look at the results for each person, shown in Exhibits 7–3 and 7–4.

The results are consistent for both groups: those who began with the week of late meals, and those who began with the early meals. The advantage of early meals is clear in the case of virtually every individual.

These differences may not seem great to you at first. Most bathroom scales cannot measure accurately within a pound or two. And people themselves—even the volunteers in this experiment—could not necessarily sense such changes over a short period of time.

"We might not have noticed the changes," said one person, "if we had not been using very accurate scales, weighing ourselves several times a day."

The 2.25 pounds-per-week advantage of early meals may not even sound sensational unless considered over a longer period of time. It would mean a weight loss of about 9 pounds per month while eating as much as 2000 calories at one meal a day on this experimental diet. By comparison, the Body Clock Diet provides fewer calories per day (1200 to 1600, depending on body size) for deliberate weight loss, and allows three meals a day plus daytime snacks for a more agreeable pattern of health, nutrition and comfort.

Results of the weight-loss experiment were reported in several articles and papers at scholarly conventions. One of the first papers was presented at the 10th International Congress on Nutrition in Kyoto, Japan, in August 1975.

Modestly, the Minnesota team states the extraordinary results in a straightforward fashion that hardly signals the importance of the discovery: "When the daily food allotment (2000 calories) was consumed for one week as breakfast, seven subjects lost weight, while if the same amount of food was consumed as an evening meal these same subjects showed either a smaller loss or a gain in weight."

The Minnesota medical labs did not limit their work to the one formal experiment with seven people, but continued the experiment.

J. J., a young woman, trim at 114 pounds, went through the two weeks, having early meals for a week, then late meals, with only 1500 calories a day. She lost 2 pounds with the early meals and gained 1 pound with the late meals. That is good supporting evidence.

The Results Are Verified and Confirmed

So exciting were these findings that I as well as other scientists became interested in verifying the conclusions and continuing the research. When the results are extremely important, scientists quite commonly reanalyze one another's data to ensure that there has been no mistake. One of the scientists was a psychologist, Professor Ed Hirsch, now at Mount Holyoke College in Massachusetts. He analyzed the data and confirmed the same conclusion: When the subjects ate 2000 calories a day as breakfast, they lost weight, but the same number of calories per day as dinner caused them to gain.

Remember, all volunteers ate the same number of calories each day whether it was the week of late meals or early meals. The

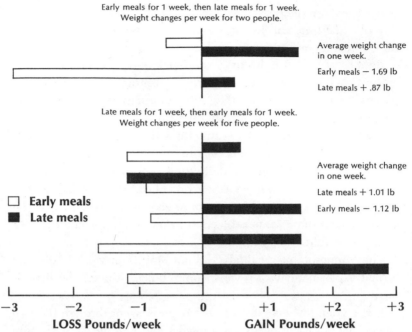

Early meals for 1 week, then late meals for 1 week.
Weight changes per week for two people.

Average weight change
in one week.

Early meals − 1.69 lb

Late meals + .87 lb

Late meals for 1 week, then early meals for 1 week.
Weight changes per week for five people.

□ **Early meals**
■ **Late meals**

Average weight change
in one week.

Late meals + 1.01 lb

Early meals − 1.12 lb

−3   −2   −1   0   +1   +2   +3
LOSS Pounds/week   **GAIN Pounds/week**

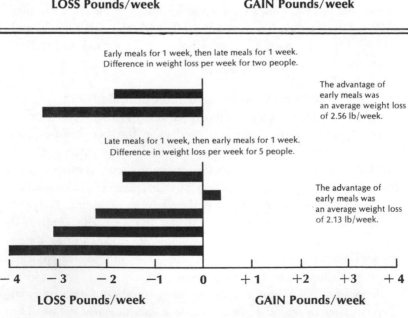

Early meals for 1 week, then late meals for 1 week.
Difference in weight loss per week for two people.

The advantage of
early meals was
an average weight loss
of 2.56 lb/week.

Late meals for 1 week, then early meals for 1 week.
Difference in weight loss per week for 5 people.

The advantage of
early meals was
an average weight loss
of 2.13 lb/week.

−4   −3   −2   −1   0   +1   +2   +3   +4
LOSS Pounds/week   **GAIN Pounds/week**

LOSING WEIGHT BY EATING EARLY

Exhibit 7-3. Eating their meals early, people lost an average of 1.28 lb in a week. Eating their meals late, the same people gained 1 lb in a week—though the menu was exactly the same and contained 2000 calories a day.

people were not particularly overweight at all, and the diet was intended to keep them just the way they were. There was no deliberate dieting here. The only interest was to determine the effects of eating food at different times in the day. And so important were these confirmed findings that the academic paper was co-authored by a total of fourteen scientists and technicians!

While the main organizer of the team was Franz Halberg, M.D., the experimental work, documentation and proof has been carried out by people with a wide variety of skills. Included was Erhard Haus, M.D., Ph.D., Professor of Pathology at the University of Minnesota and chairman, Department of Anatomical and Clinical Pathology, St. Paul-Ramsey Hospital. Also, there was Professor F. Goetz, another member of the medical faculty at the University of Minnesota.

Of the other co-authors, several were from among the volunteers themselves. Many of our volunteers in this kind of work are scientists and professionals. They simply get interested and want to help. One told me, "You get caught up in the study of body rhythms when you find out how important it is in your own body and your own life."

This particular study was a milestone in the study of nutrition and human biology, the first time such results had been reported in the United States. Appropriately, the National Institutes of Health served as local sponsor for this professional meeting, the 12th Conference of the International Society for Chronobiology,

Exhibit 7-4. Eating their meals early, people lost 2.34 lb a week more than when they ate their meals late. The menu was exactly the same and contained the same 2000 calories a day. No one was even trying to lose weight!

in Washington, D. C., in August 1975. The title of this multi-authored paper was actually shorter than the list of all the authors. They called it, "Body weight change during one week on a single daily 2000-calorie meal consumed as breakfast or dinner."

Knowledge of the earlier study was the background upon which we worked when a larger research team was formed to conduct a more complete, definitive study of the effect of breakfast and dinner calories. We worked fast. By the time Dr. Hirsch and his colleagues presented their scientific paper in Washington, D.C., we were ready with results on a whole new experiment that could be reported at the very same Conference.

We Plan a New and Larger Experiment . . .

The purpose of the new experiment was much broader and more comprehensive. It would include many aspects of food preferences, food consumption patterns, and body rhythms, as well as changes in body weight. The study was to last four months with twenty-three volunteers at two different medical centers: New Britain General Hospital and the Minnesota Medical School in Minneapolis. Both men and women would be included and their ages would range from the late teens to the mid-fifties. Mostly, they were staff professionals or students. None was unusually overweight and they might be taken as physically representative of a cross-section of the general population.

Financial support and some of the scientific expertise came from the government's Pioneering Research Laboratories at Natick, Massachusetts. There, both Dr. Harry L. Jacobs, Chief of Psychology, and Dr. S. David Bailey, head of the Food Science Laboratories, saw the opportunity for scientific breakthrough on several fronts. They chose one of their top men, Dr. R. Curtis Graeber, to head up the effort, and asked me to advise on the design of the experiment and to help plan the analysis of data. We were to work with Dr. Halberg at the University of Minnesota Medical School, and with Howard Levine, M.D., of New

Exhibit 7–5. Experimental plan to determine the effects of early versus late meals.

EXPERIMENT BEGINS

EAT ANYTIME All 23 People Adjustment Period People become adjusted to available food choices and to tests for body rhythms conducted by each person every few hours of every day. This includes body weight, blood pressure, temperature, pulse, self-ratings of mood and vigor, task-performance tests, and grip strength of each hand.	**4 WEEKS**

⬇

EAT ANYTIME All 23 People Baseline Period For comparison of the weight changes that might occur with different mealtimes in later weeks.	**2 WEEKS**

Measures of Body Rhythms from blood & urine.

⬇   ⬇   ⬇

6 WEEKS

EAT ANYTIME 5 People Control group for continuing baseline of normal weight variation.	**EARLY MEALS** 9 People Average weight loss 1.78 lb./week	**LATE MEALS** 7 People* Average weight loss 1.19 lb./week	**3 WEEKS**

Measures of Body Rhythms from blood & urine.

⬇   ⬇

	LATE MEALS Average weight gain .59 lb./week	**EARLY MEALS** Average weight loss 2.47 lb./week	**3 WEEKS**

END OF EXPERIMENT
Advantage of Early Meals

2.37 lb./week   1.28 lb./week

1.83 lb./week Average

* Of the original nine people in this group, two dropped out due to other commitments.

Britain General Hospital in Connecticut, both pioneers in the field.

At the Natick Labs, the interest was primarily in seeing if what people said they liked as food was what they would eat, and whether people could give you a fairly accurate idea of how often they would like to eat different foods. Food preferences are being assessed all the time, not only by the government, but also by food manufacturers. The U.S. government is, after all, one of the biggest buyers of food in the world.

We were to survey our volunteers' food preferences but also then monitor all of the food they ate, and their body-weight changes throughout each day. Every last morsel of food eaten was to be recorded in a diary we called the "food log." We could also calculate the nutritional value of the food they ate, check on how well they liked it when they actually ate it, and keep a record of when they ate it. In the end, there wasn't much we didn't know about their food preferences and eating behavior.

Several times a day, the volunteers were to weigh themselves so that we knew the daily fluctuation in their weights and could readily discern any trend to gain or lose. All of this was over a twelve-week period, long enough to make sure we had really meaningful data to draw our conclusions from. The overall experimental plan is shown in Exhibit 7–5.

The effect of different mealtimes was tested during a six-week period, rather than only two weeks, as in the earlier experiment. For each person in the test groups, there were three weeks eating only one daily meal as big breakfast and three weeks eating only a big dinner each day. Restricting the meals to one a day was admittedly an extreme regimen, only intended to magnify the effect of eating at different hours.

Half of the people started with the three weeks of big breakfasts and then had the three weeks of big dinners. The other half followed the procedure in the opposite order. This "crossover" design of experiment allows us to take into account any effect there might be in the order of following each diet. We expected, correctly, it turned out, that people would gain weight (or lose less) eating the dinners and lose more weight eating their daily meals at breakfast.

We had another group of volunteers who went through the whole six weeks eating whenever they liked. This would serve as a "control group," just as a basis of comparison. We would not expect them to gain or lose much weight, and that, in fact, is what happened.

People Could Eat as Much as They Liked

A person could eat as much as he or she liked, choosing freely among all the foods provided. This was a departure from the earlier experiment that told volunteers exactly what to eat, with a fixed level of calories. Here we now had a situation closer to "real life."

The meals could be taken anywhere, at home or at work; it did not matter except that the participants were to record that information. They also had to choose from supplies of food that were provided. In all, there was a good selection, with a wide choice of foods that might be typically available in a supermarket, shown in Exhibit 7–6. None of these were diet foods in the sense of having a reduced number of calories.

Remember that the volunteers were not trying to lose weight, and the available foods were not selected with that in mind.

Any leftovers were to be weighed and recorded, though portions had been sized so that in most cases the volunteers cleaned their plates. No doubt, it was less trouble for them to finish the portion than to have to weigh the leftovers.

With each thing they ate, each time they ate it, they would give it a rating for how well they liked or disliked it and record on a one-to-five scale how hungry they had been. They also noted whether they were eating alone or in company, checked off how hurried or relaxed they were at the time, and marked down the time of day when they began to eat.

For those on the restricted mealtimes, breakfast had to begin within an hour of rising and dinner could take place anytime in the evening after 6:00 P.M. There was to be no snacking and no

Exhibit 7–6. Foods provided free to volunteers, to choose as they liked. They could eat as much as they liked at a meal, and nothing on the list is particularly low in calories. None of the volunteers had any plans to lose weight, nor were they encouraged to. They were allowed to eat part of a portion if they weighed the leftovers so an accurate count could be kept of the calories consumed.

(Calories shown in parentheses.)

MAIN ENTRÉES

Beef burgundy	(320)	Ham & eggs	(335)
Beef sirloin	(316)	Sliced ham	(312)
Ham & omelet	(214)	Turkey loaf	(344)
Sausage & omelet	(391)	Beefsteak	(304)
Salisbury steak	(429)	Spaghetti beef chunks	(520)
Swiss steak	(294)	Pork slices	(320)
French-fried shrimp	(275)	Beef with sauce	(303)
Roast turkey	(197)	Chicken	(341)
Beans & franks	(396)	Tuna	(286)
Beans & meatballs	(517)	Beef slices & potato	(414)

STARCHES & VEGETABLES

Noodles	(118)	Mashed potato	(72)
Potato logs	(161)	Sweet potato	(165)
String beans	(18)	Peas & carrots	(28)
Peas	(46)	Mixed vegetables	(60)
Rice	(101)		

FRUITS, DESSERTS & SWEETS

Apple slices	(49)	Coconut-chocolate disk	(185)
Pineapple	(178)	Chocolate fudge disk	(203)
Apricots	(213)	Vanilla chocolate wafer	(216)
Pears	(182)	Chocolate nut roll	(339)
Peaches	(194)	Pecan cake roll	(448)
Applesauce	(219)	Fruit cake	(539)
Fruit cocktail	(188)	Crackers	(128)
Sweet chocolate wafer	(289)		

Instant coffee and cocoa were provided free. Other foods and beverages allowed but not provided were: sliced white bread with margarine spread, skim milk, low-calorie soda, tea, and, of course, water.

excessive dawdling over the meal. Between meals, they could have as many calorie-free drinks as they liked. In fact they were encouraged to drink a lot of fluids to help eliminate body waste.

All this sounds very detailed and restrictive, and it was. We had to control many of the things that could vary and possibly cause a gain or loss of weight. At the same time, we wanted to have the situation of people eating a varied, fairly free-choice menu, in their regular living environment. In other words, we wanted to simulate the situation of the average adult so that we could generalize about the results as they might affect the general public.

Although we provided lots of variety, it was apparently not enough. Normally, people may eat the same limited fare of their own choice, but it is another thing to have that choice limited by someone else. The only store-bought foods they could add were sliced bread, milk, and calorie-free drinks. Any candies, desserts, or other frills had to be those provided. Our brave subjects gave up all alcohol, for otherwise the caloric content would have been too hard to figure to the precision we needed. For the same reason, they had to avoid certain snacks or side dishes that are sometimes the spice of life. Potato chips and peanuts, anchovies and olives, ice cream and cookies, pie and doughnuts—all these were forbidden so that we could be sure of the nutrient and caloric content of absolutely everything that was eaten.

The volunteers worked at their regular jobs and lived at home or in college facilities. There was also the chore of weighing oneself six times or so a day, and taking other self-measurements such as blood pressure, temperature, and tests for mental-physical coordination, response time and accuracy. All that, and then the periodic days spent giving samples of blood and urine every four hours of one day, under medical supervision.

The volunteers are the heroes of this story, and it is well to assess what they were proving—that is, what was the essential difference between this experiment and the earlier, smaller one with a fixed diet of 2000 calories a day.

People were much less regimented as to what they could eat,

and were not at all limited as to how much they could eat or where they could eat it. This is closer to the "real life" situation of the average person.

We had many more volunteers in on the experiment, twenty-three instead of seven, and some of them were slated to have no mealtime restrictions at all. They would serve as a "control group" so that we could monitor "normal" eating patterns and their effect on body weight and body chemistry.

We had baseline measures of each person's normal caloric intake and weight trends for two weeks prior to the test periods of mealtime restrictions.

The new experiment lasted much longer, three times as long, to make sure that the weight changes were not just temporary.

The new experiment was conducted at two widely separated cities, Minneapolis and New Britain. It is always reassuring when scientific results emerge from more than one research center, especially if the work is going to break totally new ground and root out some old, well-established ideas about what makes us fat and what makes us thin.

So much for the background of the experiment. Now let us look at the results.

During the two weeks of the baseline period, when the volunteers could eat anytime and as much as they wished, no one gained or lost much weight. That is what we expected. When you average all the volunteers together, there was only a minimal weight loss of 1 pound over the two weeks. That is just natural variation.

The control group of six people continued to eat when they liked for another three weeks, and gained back a pound. Nothing surprising there. But those people who ate their meals early lost an average of 1.78 pounds per week. Those who ate their meals late in the day lost 1.19 pounds per week. So far, our theory is confirmed. (See Exhibit 7–5.)

What about the second three weeks? As expected, the control group weight stayed about the same, a slight increase of ½ pound. The others were now on the alternate meal plan, switching their heavy meal to the other part of the day. Eating early meals, people lost 2.47 pounds per week. The people now eating their meals late gained at the rate of .59 pounds per week. Absolutely everyone had lost substantial weight with early meals, and only two people failed to gain weight when they ate late. Remember, people could eat as much as they liked.

Everyone Lost Substantial Weight

Individual results for each person are shown in Exhibit 7–7. This shows the *difference*, for each person, between his or her weight change with early meals and the weight change with late meals. In effect, this is the relative advantage of early meals. It amounts to an overall advantage of almost 2 pounds a week during a total of six weeks.

We might rush to say that the theory is finally proved. But there is still one matter to be settled. Maybe people just ate more food when they ate their heavy meal in the evening. Maybe that increase in calories could explain the difference. That was one of the first things I was asked when I presented the results to a Columbia University Medical School seminar on October 22, 1976.

It is true that people could eat as much as they liked, and they generally ate less when they ate their meals earlier. I talked to a few of the volunteers and they told me, "We just didn't feel so hungry when we ate the early meals. It's hard to explain. You just don't feel like eating so much."

Now, nutritionists figure that 3500 calories of food eaten makes a difference of about 1 pound in your body weight, on the average. Because we know exactly what people ate, we can adjust their weight-loss figures to take into account any change in the number of calories consumed. Let us see what that shows.

After adjusting for the differences of calories, we find that people had an average weight-loss advantage of 1 pound a week when they ate their meals early rather than late. That is the dif-

83

Exhibit 7–7. Eating as much as they liked, people lost weight when they ate their meals early. Compared to late meals, early meals gave an advantage of 1.9-lb. weight loss per week, and no one was even trying to lose weight!

Early meals for 3 weeks, then late meals for 3 weeks. Differences in weight loss per week for nine people.

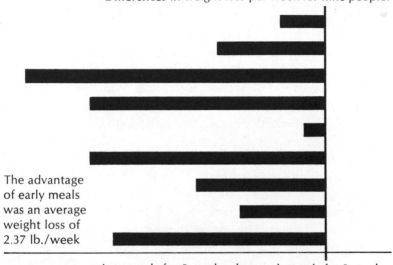

The advantage of early meals was an average weight loss of 2.37 lb./week

Late meals for 3 weeks, then early meals for 3 weeks. Differences in weight loss per week for seven people.

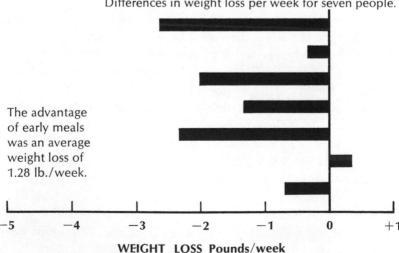

The advantage of early meals was an average weight loss of 1.28 lb./week.

−5   −4   −3   −2   −1   0   +1

WEIGHT LOSS Pounds/week

ference between what they lost with the early meals and what they gained or lost with the late meals, all adjusted for differences of caloric consumption. The effect was the same for the two groups that tested the different mealtimes in opposite order. We had to prove that. That is why we used the "crossover" design and why I show the results separately for each group of people at each stage of the experiment.

Such an Extraordinary Conclusion

We went further in our analyses, so our official government report reveals a much greater effect of early meals. The timing of the meals was shown to be about twice as important as the number of calories eaten. This conclusion was based on computer analyses of the daily weight changes and the number of calories eaten each day. Together, calories consumed and the timing of the meals explained most (57 percent) of the variation in weight changes. But the timing of the meals explained twice as much of the variation as the number of calories did. Because this is such an extraordinary conclusion, I must back it up with Exhibit 7–8.

There you have it. That is the evidence. It is all detailed in the official government report, "Human Eating Behavior: Food Preferences, Consumption Patterns, and Biorhythms," by R. C. Graeber, R. Gatty, F. Halberg, and H. Levine (published by the Pioneering Research Laboratories in Natick, Massachusetts 01760). Along with articles in the professional journals, that should satisfy scientists and medical doctors who would like to confirm our findings from a technical point of view.

Already, some professional people have been exposed to the new concepts. Early results were rushed to the annual meetings of the International Society for Chronobiology in Washington, D.C., in August of 1975. There, Dr. Harry L. Jacobs, chief psychologist at the Natick Labs, and six of our colleagues told the story for the first time in public. Within a matter of months, psychologists in New York were hearing, "You are when you eat," a further report by Drs. Graeber and Halberg at the Eastern Psychological Association. The excitement was spreading.

Quickly, the popular news media picked up the story. The *National Enquirer* printed a front-page story and *Moneysworth* magazine soon followed, getting the message out to the people. Soon, there were phone calls and letters from all across the country. Weight-loss dieting was being revolutionized, and the ground was laid for a sensible way to apply this new principle in the Body Clock Diet. Staying within the bounds of balanced nutrition and the right amount of exercise, people can now control their weight by controlling when they eat as well as what they eat.

Exhibit 7–8. In explaining weight changes, the timing of meals was twice as important as the number of calories. Together, these two factors explain most of the variation in people's weights during the six-week test period.

Explanation for Weight Change	Amount of Weight Variation Explained
Effect of when the meals were eaten	47%
Effect of the number of calories eaten	24%
Loss of information because those two factors are somewhat related	− 14%
Mealtime and number of calories considered together	57%
Other causes not included in this analysis (such as calorie-free beverages, changes in the amount of physical activity)	43%
All causes	100%

Technical note: These are the results of regression analysis, showing the partitioning of the variance, based on all 21 subjects for which data were available, including the control group as well as both test groups.

8

YOUR BODY IS REGULATED LIKE A CLOCK

Like virtually all living things, human beings go through a daily cycle. Throughout the day and the night major changes are underway, some very apparent, some subtle and unnoticed. This cycle of most body processes is repeated each day in much the same way. From hour to hour you are a different person, although from day to day there is little change unless other rhythms intercede, such as the monthly sexual cycle. Your body is primarily regulated like a twenty-four-hour clock. Longer-term changes are usually more gradual, such as the changes of the seasons or the effects of aging.

On some level you have always known this. You get sleepy about the same time each night, and you wake up at about the same time each morning. Your breakfast habits are about the same each morning, as are your toilet habits—going to the bathroom, getting ready for work, eventually having lunch. Your life is heavily scheduled not only by society, your employer, or your family, but also by your own body needs, feelings, and preferences.

Even a child knows when it is best to ask a favor of the parents, or when they are likely to say no. A wife gets to feel how differently her husband will react at different times to the same request. Curious, that on some level we know this yet we seem to ignore it in much of our daily life. It must be a matter of getting in touch with our feelings, and seeing that some of them are biologically determined by the phases of our internal rhythms.

We Are All Ruled by Our Hormones

Men speak of women as being ruled by their hormones; little do they suspect that they are equally governed by the chemistry of their bodies and minds. We tend to forget that we are biological animals, guided and even limited by the functioning of our bodies in all their physical and mental aspects.

We seem to forget that our body machine is constantly going through rhythmic processes and that we are not all exactly in phase with each other. Our arguments and misunderstandings may be based as much on body chemistry as any differences over the objective issues.

Sometimes, when we feel out of sorts, we are not in phase with ourselves. The rhythms are upset, or are adjusting to disturbances, such as illness, work fatigue, lack of sleep or food, stress, or travel across time zones that changes the length of our day. Have you ever thought of travel in that way? Traveling west, with the sun, we lengthen our day and our body may take several days to get back into synchronization. It takes just a little while longer to adjust to eastward travel, which moves against the sun and the passage of time. That is what is meant by "jet lag."

In air travel, this was first discerned by my father, Harold Gatty, and Wiley Post, who flew around the world in 1931 in eight days, in a plane called the *Winnie Mae* (now exhibited at the Smithsonian Institution in Washington, D.C.). But even before then, seafarers had noticed it and so had early travelers on the trans-Siberian railroad. Without regular sunrise and sunset to help set the interior clock, the body gets out of phase. For example, the body can no longer adapt as well to changes in outside temperature. Normally, when the room gets colder, your body generates more heat to maintain its regular temperature cycle. "Under continuous light," says Dr. Martin Moore-Ede at Harvard Medical School, "the body can't deal with external challenges anymore." He happened to prove that with gray-and-yellow squirrel monkeys, but we have good reason to believe it is true of people, too.

As individuals, we are all somewhat different from one another. We would do well to come to know our own rhythms within the day, recognize them (not fight them!), and become familiar with the natural rhythms of the people around us.

For example, some people are perky, efficient, and energized in the morning and fade toward the end of the day. We call these people "larks," in contrast to "owls," who come to life much later in the day. We have to understand that there is nothing wrong with this. It is just the way we are and it is best to accept it. Then we might be more understanding and more gentle with ourselves, and with others, too.

What a Typical Day Is Like

No one person is just like another, and these individual differences are now being measured by scientists. In general, though, people have a lot in common with each other when it comes to basic rhythms. It would be chaos if we were all different, so let us look at what is going on inside the typical person during a typical day, assuming bedtime around 11:00 P.M. and waking up about 7:00 A.M.

A lot is going on while you are still asleep. Maybe half an hour before waking, your digestive juices are about to be primed by a mounting level of chloride in the blood. Through a buffered action, the chloride ion becomes involved in the generation of stomach acids and of the enzyme (amylase) which breaks down and helps in the digestion of carbohydrates. Your body is getting ready for breakfast! Chloride also helps indirectly in the regulation of the acidity or alkalinity of your body, a vital indicator of health and well-being.

Stirring in the early hours are the adrenal glands, which prep you for the coming activities of the day and help regulate many functions of your body and mind. These glands are even more powerful, more persistent, than the more obvious sex glands, which stir to action at about the same time, as you are beginning to wake.

Both male and female hormones are rising fast in the early morning. The man has erections and the woman is potentially more interested and responsive. When most people are groping for the alarm clock, their bodies would have them groping for each other. Our social schedule expects us to romance mostly in the evening, but our bodies are trying to tell us something different.

Most of us fail to recognize that both male and female sex hormones (testosterone and estrogen) peak in the morning. You might say that people need sex before they need a cup of coffee or tea. And tea, by the way, gives the body a greater lift in the morning than it will in the evening. The tea is the same but your body is different at the later hour.

The male hormone, testosterone, also present in small amounts in women, serves a very different purpose: aside from its sexual relevance, it can play a role in the body's utilization of protein. Its morning peak may be telling us something about when the body can most efficiently use protein in our diet—namely, at breakfast.

It comes as a surprise to many people that male sex hormones have a weekly rhythm, as well as a daily one. Given a "normal" work week and social schedule, men are primed with more testosterone on Saturdays especially, but also on Wednesdays, than on other days of the week. Testosterone in the blood bottoms out on Sunday, quite probably because our social customs and sexual behavior induce us to make love by the weekly calendar.

Many men do not know that they, as well as women, have a monthly cycle in their sex hormones. How insensitive we are not to notice that! True, the outward signs are not obvious. One of the very subtle signs is that a man's beard grows more at one time of the month, the beard being a secondary sexual feature related to the flow of the male hormones.

If you are choosing a vacation time, a romantic interlude, or an evening date, why not go when your own body is attuned to what you expect of it, or hope for it?

Many women recognize that their interest in sex rises at the time of oncoming menstruation. If we may judge from a sample of thirty women, checked out over seventy lunar months, their interest is high on the fourth to the seventh day of the cycle, a week or so before ovulation. It recedes slowly over the next fifteen days, but reaches another peak just a couple of days before menstruation. Other studies indicate that their orgasms are most likely to occur around the middle of the menstrual cycle, the time of greatest fertility.

You may not be one to keep records, and certainly it is not good to become overly self-conscious, if that will inhibit you. Yet you can measure your cycle of sexual interest on a scale from zero to seven, from "no interest at all in sex" to "extremely interested in sex" (see Exhibit 8–1). This is simplest if it is done routinely at the same time each day. To check on the morning effect, just rate yourself several times throughout the day, and into the night hours, as frequently as possible, until you fall asleep. You can record your self-ratings on a form you make up (Exhibit 8–2). That also has space for other self-measurements that I will describe.

A man should also jot down when he makes love, for that will temporarily reduce his interest in sex. A discreet "SA" for "sex act" was the symbol used by male volunteers in one experiment. Woman, of course, is not burdened by such limited ability. A very preliminary pilot study suggests that for women, the sex act may actually increase desire—it whets the appetite, so to speak. It is rather like feeding a fire, and it is hard to know where it would end if carried to an extreme. In fact, it seems limited only by physical fatigue, soreness, or possible boredom. There are, after all, other interesting things to do in life.

If a man keeps the records for over a year, he is likely to find that his best month is in the fall, at least in the Northern Hemisphere. A man's fancy may turn to love in the early months of spring. That is all right for courting. It is not so good for performance. By May, his sex hormones are reaching an annual low that will perk up through the summer months to reach their peak in the late fall, sometime between September and November. If it is any consolation, he may be grateful he is not a caribou. The male caribou peaks around the same month of the year, but then that's it. The rest of the year, his hormones all but disappear.

You and I are certainly not caribou, but we just might be Eskimos. Several scientists have noted that Eskimos were sexually indifferent to each other all year, until the sun came in spring. We are told that they opened the season with five days of orgy, "an epidemic of venery, when wives and husbands are exchanged with becoming grace and good intentions," as reported by Dr. Cook as early as 1897.

To a greater or lesser extent, we all hibernate sexually, depending on how close we are to the polar regions. Menstruation itself apparently recedes during the long and dark winter months of the polar climes. Down under, in my own home country of Australia, the seasons are reversed compared with the northern half of the world. Summer comes in December and winter is in July and August. It takes quite a while for your body to adjust if you move around between the Northern Hemisphere and the Southern Hemisphere. In contrast to east–west travel, there may be no noticeable jet lag with north–south travel, but the annual autumnal peak in testosterone will have to adjust to the different seasons. This could have a small effect on sexual performance and the degree to which your body rebuilds muscle tissue, or stores fat, from the protein food that you eat. (As I mentioned earlier, testosterone may promote ability for sex but it also promotes protein utilization or metabolism.) In the tropical lands, we believe that seasonal sex hormone swings are somewhat muted. Theoretically, the people there should have a more

Exhibit 8–1. Self-rating scales to be checked off every couple of hours every day, to trace daily patterns of ups and downs. Rate yourself for a few weeks and note the rhythmic changes during a typical day for your interest in sex, and your mood and vigor.

YOUR BODY IS REGULATED LIKE A CLOCK

MOOD

1. depressed, "blue"
2. somewhat depressed
3. slightly less cheerful than usual
4. usual state
5. slightly more cheerful than usual
6. quite cheerful
7. happy, elated

HUNGER

1. not at all hungry
2. indifferent to food
3. somewhat hungry
4. definitely hungry
5. extremely hungry

VIGOR

1. inactive, tired
2. somewhat tired
3. slightly less active than usual
4. usual state
5. slightly more active than usual
6. quite active
7. active, full of pep

INTEREST IN SEX

1. no interest at all in sex
2. definitely less interested than usual
3. slightly less interested than usual
4. usual state
5. slightly more interested than usual
6. definitely more interested than usual
7. extremely interested in sex

The rating scales for mood and vigor are from an article in *The Physiology Teacher*, Jan. 1972, by Franz Halberg, M.D., and colleagues, published by the American Physiological Society. There are the same scales we used in our study of food habits and body rhythms.

steady capacity for sex, and for protein metabolism, without such strong changes from season to season.

Synchronize as a Loving Couple

If you wish to synchronize as a loving couple, you might think of shifting the menstrual cycle to match a man's cycle. We don't know yet how to shift the man's cycle, but the question for women has been better studied. Physicist Edmond Dewan proposed one method at the Rock Reproductive Clinic in Boston. His wife and a group of women showed that when they slept under the indirect light of a 100-watt bulb on the fourteenth to seventeenth nights of the cycle (counting from the first day of menstruation), their ovulation slowly synchronized to those days, as if the bulb were an artificial moon. Birth control pills can also be used to shift the cycle slowly by taking the pill for one day more or less than the twenty usually prescribed. With drugs, though, everyone ought to be super-cautious and have the advice of a medical specialist.

Back To Our Daily Routine

But enough on sex, and back to our daily routine. We are hardly out of bed yet. You will want to go to the bathroom, not just because you are now awake to do it, but because (among other things) the lack of vasopressin in your system will not let you delay. That hormonal cycle is changing and will be felt as pressure. Urine flow, however, will reach a much larger volume later, around 3:00 P.M. It is not only a simple response to how much you drink and when, but a daily rhythm that determines when it will push you toward the bathroom.

You probably also have a customary hour for voiding food waste, as well as urine. When we are healthy this is rhythmically regular, on a daily basis. We speak of being "regular" when there is no constipation. Being irregular is being out of synch with oneself. We all know that our body is healthy when it is regular and that there shouldn't be any dependence on laxatives. Some

Exhibit 8–2. To determine some of your own daily body rhythms, you can keep a record of your own self-measurements taken every couple of hours of each day, from waking in the morning to going to sleep at night. Adapt your own form for those measures that interest you. Include blood pressure, finger counting test (page 102–103, and the Sums Test (page 104) if you have the necessary equipment.

DAY OF WEEK. . . . . DATE. . . . .

Local time	Oral Temp.*	Pulse	Mood	Vigor	Hunger	Interest in sex	S. A.	Comments†
. . . . . .	. . . . . .	. . . . .	. . . .	. . . .	. . . . .	. . . . .	. . . .	. . . .
. . . . . .	. . . . . .	. . . . .	. . . .	. . . .	. . . . .	. . . . .	. . . .	. . . .
. . . . . .	. . . . . .	. . . . .	. . . .	. . . .	. . . . .	. . . . .	. . . .	. . . .
. . . . . .	. . . . . .	. . . . .	. . . .	. . . .	. . . . .	. . . . .	. . . .	. . . .
. . . . . .	. . . . . .	. . . . .	. . . .	. . . .	. . . . .	. . . . .	. . . .	. . . .

* Temperature: most accurate to use is a woman's fertility thermometer, which has finer markings, up to 100°F., than the regular oral thermometer.
† Record meals such as snack, breakfast, lunch, dinner (S, B, L, D), and unusual exertion or emotional events.

95

accustom their bodies to need laxatives, thus setting up an addictive habit to be broken.

Be careful if you are shaving in the morning. Our best evidence shows that if you are going to nick yourself, it is better to do it in the evening because the blood will clot faster then. The slowest time for blood clotting seems to be around midday, with 50 percent more time needed to stop the flow. That is fine, since few of us are shaving in the middle of the day.

Your body temperature is low at the beginning of your day. It will vary a degree or more within the day, usually rising to a peak around the middle or latter part of the afternoon. Whoever told you that 98.6° Fahrenheit was a constant norm? The rhythmic pattern varies with individuals, as does most everything else. Some people's temperatures rise earlier in the day. Those are the people who are more efficient, better performers, in the morning: the "larks." "Owls" will find their temperatures rising more slowly, peaking later and bringing with it their best mental and physical abilities.

Your Energy Reserves Are Low in the Morning

Your basic energy level is very low in the morning, even if you have had a heavy meal the night before.

This basic energy that directly fuels the body is glucose, or blood sugar as it is sometimes called. You eat foods to fuel your body, but they all end up to some degree as glucose, though the various pathways and processes are different and vitally important. You need to eat protein, fat, and carbohydrate, and let the body make the glucose. Trying to short-circuit your system by eating straight glucose sugar would leave you without other vital ingredients, such as vitamins and minerals.

Usually your body has on tap only about one-fifth of an ounce of glucose in circulation, hardly more than a fifteen-minute supply—and that is the only fuel that the brain can normally use.

As a protective buffer, you have an extra supply of glucose in a more concentrated form known as glycogen, stored mainly in the liver. There, you have a few hours' supply of glucose, even as much as eighteen hours if you don't move about much.

The fat on your body, and even the flesh, is a more remote form of energy storage that can be used for calories in the absence of glucose if you stop eating long enough. Most of us have some forty days' supply of food energy put away in our body fat. If you do stop eating, you will deplete your glycogen and will start burning up calories from other parts of the body. Unless you eat protein, too much of that weight loss will come from your muscle flesh, and that isn't part of you you want to lose!

Your supplies of glycogen energy are depleted in the morning, and it may be late afternoon before they rise again to their fullest. Meanwhile, if you do not eat, you are likely to have a low energy level. You might not notice it yourself, especially if you have become accustomed to it. We are so often insensitive to our own bodies' needs. But if you eat sensibly, you will feel better. Don't take my word for it, try it! Low blood sugar brings on irritability and impatience, and is often the cause of family spats and arguments. Early morning grumpiness is a common problem that may be solved by a nutritious breakfast. A person relatively low in blood sugar and glycogen may have symptoms of depression, fatigue, anxiety and irritability, all associated with hypoglycemia, in the extreme case.

Following the changing level of blood sugar, family disputes may be rhythmically timed within the day without your even knowing why! Another time to watch for declining blood sugar is the early evening before supper. If people do not get supper when they expect it, and when their bodies need it, they may become quite disgruntled, as much because of falling blood sugar as anything else.

When our bodies sense that our blood sugar is very low, we often feel like eating something sweet—sugared doughnuts, Danish pastry, breakfast cereal with lots of sugar, toast with jam, or even candy. We get a sudden "sweet tooth," a craving for something sweet.

It is better, though, to eat nutritious foods containing vitamins and minerals, and especially those foods which have more pro-

97

tein, or even fat or starch, rather than sugar. Sugar itself contains nothing but calories. Besides being very bad for the teeth, it is too much of a jolt to the system, rather like pouring gasoline on a fire that is fading. What you want for a steady pace is protein, fat, or starch that will be transformed gently in the body to become glucose in accord with the body's own timing, regulated as it needs it.

Peaking around 10:00 A.M. will be one of the important amino acids (tyrosine) that plays a role in the conversion of food to usable forms for the body. It would be well to take advantage of that and to have eaten a fair share of your day's calories by the time the body is ready and best able to work on it.

Exercise Accentuates This Rhythm

Exercise accentuates this rhythm and so aids the conversion of food at the peak times. If you have a lot of physical or mental activity ahead during the day, it will be all the more important to start the day off with a hearty breakfast or brunch. By the latter part of the afternoon, your tyrosine level is likely to be only half as high as it is in mid-morning.

The morning level of amino acids may be raised even higher with a big, protein-rich breakfast such as a couple of eggs, or fish, meat or cheese and milk. The same meal in the evening will hardly raise the level at all, according to studies done at the U. S. Army Medical Research Institute in Frederick, Maryland.

The body's utilization of protein leaves traces in the system: blood urea nitrogen reaches a high by late afternoon to early evening. And the peak in urea by-product of the protein utilization will have occurred by that time. Similarly, as a result of muscular activity, creatinine in the urine has usually peaked by midafternoon. Protein utilization, then, is not necessarily timed optimally to cope with the usual heavy evening meals.

If you are to face a stressful day, better stock up early on protein. You will need more than usual, and the same goes for sleepless nights when your job or your baby may keep you up. Both stress and wakeful nights increase your need for protein, though

98

it may take a day or more for your body to show that it is deprived. Only your doctor would know for sure, but why take chances?

Your body uses food differently during the different hours of the day. But food also tastes different at different hours. Early in the day you may be fairly good at discriminating between two different tastes, smells, or sounds. This seems related to the high level of adrenal cortical hormones in your blood, according to some authors. As the day progresses to late afternoon and early evening, you will be less able to discriminate between two levels of intensity, but you will have a keener threshold of perception.

This means that in the evening you can get the same effect by using less salt and less sweetener and you will not be able to tell the difference in amount, because you are insensitive to differences of intensity at that time. A little will seem to be as much as a lot. On the other hand, you will be much more able to tell whether or not there is *any* salt, sweetener, or other flavoring.

The same is true of hearing. In the morning it may not irritate you if the children are making a lot of noise, while in the evening the same amount of noise could drive you out of your head. In the evening you will be more readily able to tell if someone is ringing the doorbell but less able to tell if it is the front door or the back door.

Perhaps the best example is with the neighbor's television set. It rarely disturbs you in the morning because then your neighbor knows when it is too loud, and moderates it, while you can't hear low sound-levels at all. In the evening, your neighbor is almost totally insensitive to just how loud it is and you are better able to hear any sound that penetrates the wall.

The senses are different from hour to hour, and so are the reactions of your body to stimulants and drugs. Tea, we have mentioned, has more impact in the morning. So too does alcohol. Fortunately, it is not customary to drink alcohol in the morning. Alcohol at any time is a poison to the body, but strong evidence now suggests that it is much more toxic in the morning.

Headaches may not be one of your problems, but some people

have them recurrently and persistently. I have talked with people who suffer migraines from severe headaches, and it seems that each person knows when is the most likely time of the day for them to recur. What they may not know is that you can use a lighter dose of aspirin in the morning than at night to do the same job. Toward evening, the aspirin doesn't stay in circulation as long as it does in the morning.

We breathe rhythmically, of course, and though you probably never stopped to think about it, you are taking about twenty breaths per minute. With pressure and activity, that can be doubled or even tripled. As much as a quarter of the oxygen you take in will be used by the brain, so to keep a clear head it is a good idea to breathe deeply from time to time and get plenty of good ventilation. In some sense, oxygen is a kind of food for the body. There should be good, clean air and plenty of it. You will be using more of it each minute as the day progresses, but then your consumption of it will drop off rapidly after you have been asleep for about an hour. Your heart is working as a pump on about the same schedule, with a rising rate of output through the day. No, it is not just a matter of things slowing down when you sleep. Even if you stay wide awake, your breathing will slow down on schedule.

Ninety-Minute Ups and Downs

Throughout the day, you will be functioning on about a ninety-minute rhythm of ups and downs that you may never have noticed. That is, you may have never recognized the regularity of your ups and downs. Ninety minutes is about the limit of your concentration on any one thing. For a child it is about half that time. So there is good reason for your periodic pauses during the day or evening. The advice is not to push yourself. Go with the rhythms, not against them. Take your breaks when you are on a low, and catch the upswing to ride with the natural rhythms whenever you can. Ideally, you should be so in tune with your own system that you don't even think about it. It is all so natural.

YOUR BODY IS REGULATED LIKE A CLOCK

Within the day, much that you do, think, feel and sense, will be paced on that ninety-minute cycle. For some people it may average eighty-five minutes, for others 110 minutes. Your brain waves are paced on this schedule day and night. One oddity that relates to eating is that many people keep this same rhythm when it comes to putting things in their mouths. They may reach for a cigarette, bite their nails, put pencils in their mouths, or bite the end of a pen. Most importantly, it could mean eating a snack or taking a drink.

For dieters, this is a dangerous thing. That trip to the refrigerator may be prompted not by hunger in any real sense, but by the rhythmic urge for oral satisfaction. It is not very different from a baby's periodic need for a pacifier to hold in its mouth. Some of us manage by using a glass of water to hold and to sip. It is as good a solution as any. It is harmless and, in fact, you are better off taking plenty of liquids throughout the day, as long as they do not add calories. But if you can hold off the oral urge for fifteen minutes, you are likely to forget it, for the urge will pass quickly with the changing rhythms. The oral urge does not mean real hunger at all. When you know that, and know that it will pass, you can cope with it better.

Even real hunger moves in rhythms. Actual pangs of hunger feel like contractions of the stomach, telling you it is ready to receive food it is not getting. Over fifty years ago it was proved by Tomi Waada that these physical rhythms occur every ninety to one hundred minutes. We are not sure whether they occur at the same time as the oral urge. If you fed both regularly you might get very fat indeed!

The secret of control lies in always knowing that the pangs and urges will pass, as they pass their peak on rhythms, whether you feed them or not. If you can hold out for a while, you will not feel the need any more—till the next time around! On the other hand, they are as good a time as any to take your regularly planned snacks that will keep your blood sugar on a more even keel. You can keep a record of your hunger feelings in your chart (Exhibit 8–2), rating them from one to five, "not at all hungry" to "extremely hungry"; try to make sure that they are real hunger feelings and not just an urge for oral satisfaction.

As the afternoon approaches, so does your peak performance at many different mental and physical tasks. You become faster and more accurate in mental tasks. You are physically stronger. And there is better coordination between your mind and your body. That is worth knowing about! I, for one, put off some chores—and don't feel guilty about it—waiting for my peak to come. You might consider doing the same. After all, you are not a robot!

While we can generalize about people and their peak times, we are all still individuals when it comes to peaking in somewhat different ways at somewhat different times. Our big study showed people peaking from around noon to 1:00 P.M. in measures of task performance. We included both men and women from their late teens to their late fifties.

The point is not to expect your peak to be at the same time as those of our volunteers, but to realize that you have peaks and troughs and to learn when they occur for you, and for those close to you.

So far, in general, it seems that physical tasks are best performed toward afternoon. Optical reaction time is slowest in the dead of night. If the task calls for coordination of eye and hand, or requires a quick perception, late night is not the time to do it. It seems that in many ways we are at our lower levels of ability during the hours when we are usually asleep!

You Can Measure Some of Your Own Rhythms

You may want to measure yourself on some rhythms. I think, though, that many of us can sense when we are at our best. If only we would go along with our feelings and be sensitive to our natural selves! But if you do want to do some rhythmic measures, here are a few tasks to check yourself out.

You need a stopwatch for this one. Hold it in your left hand while you count the fingers of your right hand. (If you are a "leftie" do this with the opposite hand.) Hold the right hand in front of you, palm up. Count each finger by touching it with the thumb, starting with the first finger, counting down through the little finger and up again, repeating this till you get to a count of 25, when your thumb should be back at the first finger. Immediately repeat this to another count of 25 and note down how many seconds this took, accurate to one-tenth of a second. After the first few tries you will be adept at it, and I promise that you will be regularly faster or slower at certain hours of the day or night.

Of course people will think you a little odd if you do this on a bus or a train, or anywhere in public. Better to do your test in private where you will not be disturbed. However, you should do it at least six times throughout the day, preferably every couple of hours.

Perhaps arithmetic was not your favorite subject in school. Many of us, it seems, have had some bad experiences with it and have lost confidence in our ability to add a bunch of numbers together. But our ability, or lack of it, is actually a sometime thing that depends on the hour of the day. You may not be as bad at arithmetic as you think you are, if you would just choose the right hour of the day to do your sums!

Here is the Sums Test we used to check on the best time for adding speed and accuracy: We use a table of random numbers, choosing a different column of fifty digits each time. You can use the table in Exhibit 8–3. Start a stopwatch, then add each pair of digits, going down the column so you end with a list of forty-nine numbers jotted down on a piece of paper. Immediately write down how much time it took you, accurate to one-tenth of a second. Your score is figured as the number of correct additions divided by the number of seconds it took you. Don't make a mistake figuring your score!

It is even easier to keep track of your pulse and your temperature. You will probably find them rising to a peak in the afternoon. All these things can be measured, though that is not at all necessary in order to follow the Body Clock Diet. Some people find it fun, and in Minnesota, huge numbers of high school children have had classroom projects to keep track of their basic rhythms. If they can do it, you can do it too!

Speaking casually, we often refer to our heart as our "ticker," in recognition of its clocklike rhythms. Heart rate is, of course, one of the basic rhythms, as is blood pressure. Blood pressure can be measured at home, and self-measurement kits are sold for this purpose. They can be used safely if one follows the directions carefully. Peak blood pressure comes after midday. Average normal readings run 110 to 120 for the pumping pressure (systolic pressure) and around 70 or 80 for the pressure at rest (diastolic pressure), although a higher reading can certainly be quite normal, as with elderly people, for example. During the day you will find a swing of about four to seven in the readings. Of course exercise, anxiety or arguments can temporarily raise the pressure, so the readings ideally should be done under similar conditions each time to plot the daily rhythm. All in all, you have about ten pints of blood, and it will be recycled a thousand times during the day. The heart is an impressive piece of rhythmic machinery and deserves your respect.

Remember, we are not trying to diagnose ourselves when we take our own blood pressure. We are only trying to check on the rhythms during the day; however, such records may help your doctor and alert him to problems. Leave it to your doctor to tell you if your blood pressure is too high, and what importance your blood pressure reading has to your own health.

Exhibit 8–3. The Sums Test: This is a test you can do yourself to find when during the day or night you are best at doing your sums. Going down a column of numbers, add each pair of digits—in the first column, for example, 7 + 2, 2 + 6, 6 + 7. Jot your answers down to check when you finish. Your score is the number of correct additions divided by the number of seconds you took to finish the column, accurate to 1/10 second. You will need a stopwatch. And figure your score correctly!

YOUR BODY IS REGULATED LIKE A CLOCK

Choose a different column each time you test yourself.

7	4	8	5	4	4	5	6	6	3	0	2
2	2	1	5	8	4	7	8	8	1	2	5
6	0	4	6	6	1	1	0	3	9	0	6
7	2	0	7	3	5	1	3	7	2	0	1
9	6	9	0	0	4	1	7	2	5	1	0
6	2	0	1	2	5	4	3	3	4	4	3
0	5	7	3	4	0	3	5	4	6	3	2
8	9	8	9	6	3	3	3	8	0	7	5
7	3	9	1	4	7	6	0	6	8	7	3
6	3	5	8	6	3	5	8	4	1	7	2
6	9	3	3	3	8	7	8	7	3	8	6
2	0	9	7	5	4	1	3	6	9	5	5
2	1	5	9	7	5	0	9	2	5	5	6
7	1	2	2	9	8	7	2	4	3	4	3
1	0	7	1	9	7	8	6	1	0	1	8
5	6	1	7	3	5	1	7	9	1	3	7
7	5	2	6	7	6	3	2	2	0	7	9
8	6	0	5	7	4	1	7	1	0	3	9
0	1	1	6	5	3	4	3	2	2	4	9
4	9	7	8	4	9	1	1	8	7	4	6
2	1	7	8	6	2	5	3	4	1	8	0
6	8	7	7	1	8	9	8	3	6	5	8
6	7	7	5	6	1	2	4	7	7	1	9
0	2	5	8	3	2	8	7	9	2	8	8
1	3	0	6	0	5	4	3	2	6	1	7
3	1	0	0	2	5	9	1	6	3	8	6
6	2	9	7	7	3	6	7	9	6	8	6
0	0	2	4	7	7	0	7	2	5	0	5
1	4	4	7	7	8	7	0	3	0	1	6
6	5	2	3	1	4	0	2	4	6	8	3
1	6	1	2	0	2	7	6	0	1	9	3
0	8	7	3	6	9	1	6	9	2	9	5
5	1	8	1	1	8	9	3	0	0	6	8
7	0	0	3	4	6	0	7	6	8	8	7
8	4	5	4	6	0	7	3	1	7	2	9
7	7	3	5	0	5	0	6	5	6	3	6
7	2	9	1	4	9	9	6	8	1	1	3
7	5	8	0	0	6	8	2	9	9	9	7
7	7	8	4	9	5	0	7	6	7	1	1
9	0	4	6	1	9	6	1	9	9	0	0
2	9	5	5	9	4	1	2	5	8	5	0
4	4	5	7	5	2	6	7	9	7	9	9
0	5	9	0	8	1	3	5	1	1	5	4
8	1	8	2	3	7	2	5	7	1	3	8
1	0	6	2	5	8	9	1	4	6	9	4
3	0	5	1	0	5	5	0	1	5	7	8
8	6	9	3	7	6	7	5	8	2	7	1
0	9	4	3	3	7	4	4	5	3	8	0
1	0	3	9	0	6	5	4	5	2	3	7
6	2	8	5	5	3	0	3	5	0	5	9

THE EFFECTS OF THE BODY CLOCK

We find that the rhythms of blood pressure correspond fairly closely to daily rhythms in how vigorous you feel. That can be measured simply by rating yourself on the scale going from "inactive, tired" to "active, full of pep." All seven categories of this scale are shown in Exhibit 8–1. You may be able to discern the difference it makes when you start the day with a good breakfast. We examine such changes statistically, but in many cases you can see the daily trend quite clearly by just looking at the results.

Your mood will be peaking around the same time as your vigor, by midday or sometime during the afternoon. This too can be rated by you on a rating scale that goes from "depressed, blue," to "happy, elated," shown in the same Exhibit. Rate yourself—your own vigor and mood—as often as possible during the day and evening to find your own average peak and bottom. You may find, as I did for our volunteers, that people vary: some peaked as early as noon, while others were late peakers, closer to 5:00 P.M. Maybe that is the difference between "larks" and "owls."

Besides the daily rhythms, you may expect mood swings for both men and women on a cycle of at least four weeks. Men do have a monthly (or longer) period in mood as well as in sexual hormones, though either rhythm may be affected by what else happens during the month.

Do not judge others by yourself, though. One of our volunteers, a medical doctor, told me that he didn't think the mood ratings were very useful. "The ratings are about the same each day," he said. "They hardly change from day to day. They just start rising in the morning and reach a peak around noon." I had to show him that other people had peaks quite a bit later in the day. Personally, I think it can help living and working with others if we get to know and respect our own rhythms and also the rhythms of the people around us.

If you want to know more about how to measure your own rhythms, you can get more technical instructions from the references listed for this chapter, particularly the basic study by Dr. R. C. Graeber, myself, Dr. Franz Halberg, and Dr. Howard Levine, or from an earlier article in *The Physiology Teacher* (January 1972), by Dr. Halberg and his colleagues, which we ourselves used as a first how-to-do-it manual.

Your mood and vigor are high in the afternoon and your optical reaction time is as fast as it ever becomes. Reaction time for eyesight is at its slowest around 4:00 A.M. You are usually asleep then, but even if you are awake, your responses will be slow.

Your physical strength is up during the day. We measure that with a hand-grip meter called a dynamometer. A squeeze with each hand in turn allows us to read off an index of grip strength for right and left hands. Dr. Juergen Aschoff reports the peak around noon, then a fast falloff to 3:00 P.M., a rise in the late afternoon and an extreme low during the night hours. In our research we got similar results, with high readings by 1:00 P.M.

Adrenaline is related to strength, and though that has a normal daily rhythm, it can be influenced by stress and emergencies. One of its possible effects is to suppress hunger, and it will be reaching its peak at about 2:00 P.M. A close relative, noradrenaline, is probably even more relevant to appetite, and it peaks at about the same time. Like adrenaline, noradrenaline is additionally important to us because, among its many functions, it tends to inhibit insulin secretion and to offset the fattening effects of our natural insulin. That may help explain why calories consumed early have less of a fattening effect than calories consumed late in the day.

Your energy stores of glucose are likely to be at a peak in the late afternoon, and fat-forming insulin is normally peaking around the same time. That should signal to you that you do not need much more food to maintain yourself through the relatively inactive hours of the night. It also means that insulin is there in abundance to form fat from any surplus calories you eat!

Tie a string around your finger if you have to, to avoid excess calories after mid-afternoon. Your ability to remember was probably peaking about then. Later in the day you might forget more easily that excess food means excess fat, especially if eaten late in the day, or at night.

You are already heavier in the latter part of the afternoon and will continue to be heavy into the night hours. Your weight follows a daily cycle of regular ups and downs, though your bathroom scale probably cannot read accurately enough to trace the changes. In our experiments, we used medical scales accurate to at least a couple of ounces. Of course, a couple of glasses of water can change your weight quickly, but most of us have fairly regular habits and fairly regular daily patterns in how much we weigh at any particular hour of the day or night. Through the month, a woman will also have the added weight of an additional one to four pounds of water retained at the beginning of menstruation.

The coming of darkness will stimulate a hormone, melatonin, which is thought to modify one's physical activity and, at least indirectly, influence the coming of sleep. Some scientists also believe that it also slows up the sex hormones in a child's development to maturity. They note that youngsters in the warmer climates, with longer hours of sunshine, develop to sexual maturity at an earlier age. It is even noted that in recent years, with widespread use of electric lights, girls in northern climates are coming to sexual maturity at an earlier age. The same hormone also affects skin color in response to light—the effect of tanning when you sun yourself. It is a good example of how complex our body system is, with some hormones serving several body functions that are not all yet fully understood. What they affect, and what affects them, is often crucially important and quite complicated.

In the evening, for example, your sex hormones are normally far from peaking. But you might check the barometer if you are not sure the urge or ability is there. One study reports that increased sexual activity is related to low atmospheric pressure. In future studies of body rhythms I hope to record barometric pressure as one more possible influence on the ups and downs of the day. There is already some indication that it may be related to how you feel in both health and sickness.

If you happen to suffer allergies, you may well find that they act up more in the evening hours. Allergies to penicillin, house dust, feathers, histamine, and grass pollen all seem to be concentrated in the evening hours, and asthma problems are accentuated. Also, toothache is more painful at this time, at least when prompted experimentally by a jolt of electricity.

At night, as we have said before, you become more sensitive to detection of sounds, tastes, and smell, possibly brought on by the evening's rhythmic decline in adrenal cortical hormones. Some say it may be related to changing salinity in the saliva, but we are not really sure. We do know, though, that these things vary rhythmically within the day.

At night, also, you are more resistant to infection. Counts of white blood cells reveal this, as do counts of gamma globulin, which has antibodies of immunity to viruses and bacteria.

Sleep itself will bring on the flow of the growth hormone, vital to us all, and especially to children. Among many other functions, it will help prevent your natural insulin from lowering the body's level of energy too far.

For women, menstruation will most often begin in the small hours of the morning, and the overall cycle will still be in time with a lunar cycle of 29.5 days, although individuals will vary. Conception, if it is to occur, is most likely during the three days of the full moon. Birth will normally occur 265 or 266 days later, usually in the early morning. That seems appropriate because in the natural order of things, morning is also the time most likely for death.

Our knowledge of the biological calendar and the daily biological clock has been drawn from many different studies on many different people. The hourly changes, the peaks and crests, can be somewhat different from one person to another, and we are now studying some of those differences. We know by now that any one peak may not be meaningful by itself. The important thing is to recognize the whole process of body change, involving the many related changes that can depend on each other, or affect each other.

Do not think of the hours I have given as norms your body should be following. We each march to a somewhat different drummer. How we live, work, play or sleep may well affect our rhythms. The kinds of foods we eat and when we eat them can alter some of the rhythms. We must begin by feeling, understanding, and respecting the rhythms of our own unique body clock. Most simply, it is a matter of respecting our own selves and treating ourselves well and wisely. Good health requires eating the right kind of foods at the right times, and working in accord with our body rhythms, not against them.

9

HOW MEALTIMES MODIFY YOUR BODY CLOCK

Eating actually modifies the rhythms of your body clock in many invisible but important ways that you may not know about. Both what you eat and when you eat it alter certain rhythms, and some of them relate to gaining or losing weight.

It is not only food that modifies these rhythms. The timing or duration of the light and dark parts of the twenty-four-hour day— even electric lights—also have an effect. When and how long you sleep may affect the rhythms. Physical activity also affects some rhythms, either in their timing or in the degree of their ebb and flow. And finally, some drugs may affect the rhythms. All of these things can help synchronize your body clock. Misused, they can throw you out of kilter.

We are beginning to understand the effects of food and different mealtimes through experiments and careful measurement. Some of what we know can be sketched briefly with notes on practical implications. A few of the things going on inside you will be new and unfamiliar. It is not necessary to understand them to follow the Body Clock Diet. So skip this chapter if you do not care to look inside yourself, at the complexities of what is happening. But you might just find it fascinating to see what is going on inside your body when you eat at different times of the day.

The level of your blood sugar is an indication of immediately available energy that you can use. Blood sugar, or glucose, has a daily rhythm even if you eat nothing, according to scientists Jores and Lakatua. But it is influenced by what you eat and when you eat.

Dr. Raymond Greene of London's Northern Hospital notes that eating "protein produces a slow increase in blood sugar, which persists for three or four hours ('Meat stays by you'). Carbohydrate produces a rapid rise in blood sugar followed in an hour or so by a reactive drop." The effect of eating fat is to raise the blood sugar fast, but the rapid falloff in energy is halfway between that of protein and carbohydrate, according to Dr. Greene. (See Exhibit 9–1.)

This means that for breakfast, sweet pastry, a doughnut or sugared cereal will not sustain you for long. Eating sugar or starch results in a depression of hunger and weakness within two hours. You need protein or even fat to do the job if you want to avoid a real downer, which you just might be so accustomed to that you don't even recognize it. Protein may take an hour to have much effect but it will sustain you for about four hours on a fairly steady basis. As outlined elsewhere in this book, it is a good idea to put ample protein in your breakfast, as well as in your other meals.

For a quick lift, starch carbohydrate is okay. Bread is a good choice because it has other nutrients as well as calories. Sugar is a "no-no" because it has nothing but quick-acting calories that give you a sudden lift and a sudden, hard drop, while it wrecks your teeth.

We've Been Taught to Indulge Our Sweet Tooth

It is hard to avoid sugar simply because it is used in so many processed foods that we eat daily. It is a convenient preservative for the food manufacturers and it is a relatively cheap ingredient. Also, it caters to the sweet tooth we have been taught to indulge. Unfortunately, it is found in everything from

Exhibit 9–1. A high-protein breakfast (eggs, lean meat or fish, dairy products) sustains blood sugar energy throughout the morning. A high-carbohydrate breakfast (bread, doughnuts, sugar) results in immediate energy but leads to a rapid and drastic decline in blood sugar within an hour of breakfast. The effect of a high-fat breakfast is intermediate. (Adapted from Dr. Raymond Greene, *Human Hormones,* London, 1970, p. 232.)

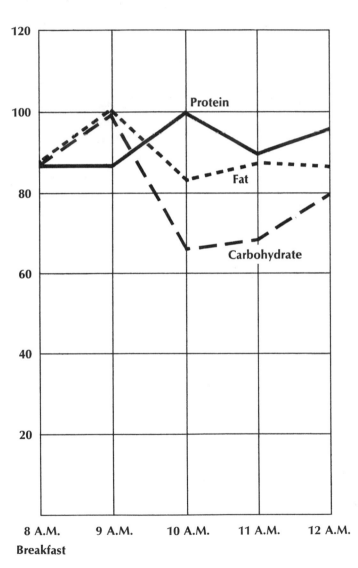

soups to salad dressings, cakes, cookies, cereals, ketchup and processed meats.

Whatever sugar you do eat, you will be better off eating it in the morning. That is when the calories will do less harm in adding to your waistline. Dr. R. J. Jarrett of London's Guy's Hospital Medical School has shown that glucose tolerance is best in the morning and worsens as the day progresses. He also found that overly plump people had a less accentuated daily rhythm of glucose tolerance, so that is all the more reason for overweight people to avoid not only excess calories in general, but sugar in particular.

Glucose tolerance is best in the morning, and actual levels of blood sugar are lower after an early meal than after late meals, a fact proved by several scientists. Glucose in the system is managed by hormonal secretions of the pancreas. One particular hormone that helps move glucose into storage is insulin, though some of us could use a little less help in that department. Bluntly stated, insulin indirectly tends to make us fat. To add insult to injury, injected insulin may also induce hunger pangs. Curiously, our natural insulin seems to be a factor in our feeling we have had enough to eat.

Unfortunately, overweight people require more insulin to offset glucose than do slender people. It is a Catch-22 situation if a person is already overweight. That is the bad news. The good news is that a little of your natural insulin goes a long way in the morning.

Natural insulin levels were far lower after early meals than late meals when volunteers ate exactly the same number of calories each day. Insulin rises after meals. With early meals, it peaked around 10:00 A.M., a time when most people are quite active. Its peak was almost three times the day's average level. After late meals it peaked at 8:00 P.M., when most people are relatively inactive. And it peaked 100 percentage points higher. Therefore evening meals may be far more fattening!

Another pancreatic hormone moderates the effect of insulin and releases stored sugars and fats. It is called glucagon and it is our friend if we are fat and want to lose weight. It is even good enough to reduce our true hunger pangs (feelings of contractions in the stomach) and help us recognize when we have had enough food. Whenever we eat, glucagon peaks about three hours after insulin does, but after early meals it rises to a relatively higher level (140 percent instead of 130 percent over the day's average). So again, we might see this as an advantage of the early meals.

The importance of all this for weight control was pointed out by a team of fourteen scientists writing in the journal *Experientia* in 1976. They included the well-known names of Professors Frederick Goetz, Franz Halberg and Erhard Haus of the University of Minnesota, and Drs. Ian D. Smith, an Australian countryman of mine from the University of Sydney, and Marion Apfelbaum from the University of Paris. They analyzed hormonal results of the early-versus-late-meal test with seven volunteers eating 2000 calories per day, in the experiment we discussed earlier.

They quite directly suggest that meal-induced changes in internal timing may contribute to the relative weight loss with early meals. They do note that the weight loss might be due to different "caloric cost" of physical activity, interacting with the timing of the meals. How it all works is not yet fully explained, but the result is clear: Relative body weight goes down when meals are eaten early. We are virtually certain that insulin and glucagon flows are basic to the explanation. We may yet find that insulin and glucagon are competing for a limited number of calories in the case of early meals, while with late meals the peaks of the two rhythms occur at more widely separated times. However, the explanation should probably not be limited to insulin and glucagon, but should include adrenaline and noradrenaline as well.

A Key Regulator of the Hormones

One of the most exciting discoveries of the past fifteen years has been the identification of one of the key regulators of hormones, according to Professor Ruth Pike of Pennsylvania State University and Myrtle Brown of the National Academy of Sciences. This compound is called cyclic AMP. Simply stated, it causes the breakdown of fat deposits in your body and it is present in every cell of your body in varying amounts through the day and night. We may think of it as countering the fattening effect of insulin. But now, what about its rhythms in relation to when you eat? The above-mentioned article in *Experientia* tells the story.

When volunteers ate early meals, the cyclic AMP (measured in the urine) peaked after the middle of the afternoon, from 3:30 to 4:30 P.M. Late meals pushed the peak earlier in the afternoon, between 12:30 and 2:30 P.M. That does not seem like a big difference perhaps, but it could be enough to show up on your bathroom scale in terms of pounds. When the diet was early meals, the cyclic AMP maintained a higher average daily level in two of the three cases studied, and it had an amplitude swing that was 50–100 percent greater than when late meals were eaten. But the story is not so simple. Other rhythms in the body are also important.

Effects of the Adrenal Glands

As many people know, adrenaline helps us mobilize ourselves for quick action and stress. In emergencies it can surge forth in astonishing amounts, increasing as much as a thousand-fold. It suppresses our hunger, reduces our insulin level and makes energy available for immediate use. It also raises the blood pressure and supplies more blood to the muscles for active use.

During a normal day adrenaline peaks about 2:00 P.M., according to Dr. Halberg's team of researchers. That is fine for a hunger-controlling, anti-fattening effect during the afternoon, but it won't help you much if you unwind in the evening with a heavy meal.

From another part of the adrenal gland come hormones that may be even more basic to weight control than adrenaline. Franz Halberg says that these "may be the pacemakers of twenty-four-hour periodic metabolism." Most people have heard of cortisone used in the treatment of arthritis, and that is one form of these hormones called corticoids. They control body processes by an indirect feedback mechanism, in contrast to the more direct mechanism of control by the central nervous system.

The flow of at least some of these hormones is affected by the timing of your meals. Some of them (the glucocorticoids) decline at night, making you more sensitive to low levels of sound, taste and smell, according to Dr. Robert Henkin and his team at the National Institutes of Health. More important to us is the fact that at least one of them (cortisol) has a lot to do with making energy reserves available for use and slowing down the formation of fat.

Cortisol peaks in the urine from about 9:30 A.M. to 2:30 P.M., following a low during the dead of night. It rises and falls as much as 30 percent over and under the twenty-four-hour daily average, according to Dr. Juergen Aschoff of the Max Planck Institute.

In our own experiment, cortisol was measured in the blood, and similar results were found, with a peak at 9:30 A.M. Late meals delayed the cortisol peak only by an hour, not enough to be of much help in coping with the calories of late meals. Also, with exclusively late meals, the average level of cortisol was lower and the rhythmic swing was dampened.

If Your Face and Hands are Puffy in the Morning

You may be one of those people who wake up feeling "puffed," with the face, fingers or other parts of the body swollen with too much overnight water retention in the tissues. You might, for instance, have trouble getting a ring off your finger without using soap or oil and a lot of pulling, twisting and tugging. Or you awaken but feel that your face hasn't; around your eyes especially, you feel puffed and swollen. Sodium is one of the main culprits in the water retention that causes this swelling (as well as in high blood pressure), and it is governed to some extent by cortisol, but mainly by the periodic flow from another adrenal hormone, aldosterone.

Aldosterone rises rapidly in the blood at the onset of sleep and reaches high concentrations during the night. Knowing this, it would seem that doctors might be able to advise patients better now as to when during the day they might indulge more freely in salt (sodium chloride) and when one could drink more liquids without getting puffed in the morning. Most of us take five times more sodium than is necessary in our diet. Almost all of us should cut down on it. But the time of day also makes a difference!

In salt it is not only the sodium that is important but also the chloride. Indirectly chloride helps to regulate the acidity of the blood. It is vital to the formation of stomach acids that hold off digestion of fats that you would rather not see added to your waistline. Also, chloride activates the enzyme that breaks down starch. With a diet of heavy dinners, blood chloride is peaking well after the middle of the night when you are asleep. With early meals, chloride rises to a crest a few hours after you wake up.

Lecithin is already known to many people for its ability to break up and dissolve fat in the body. One of its components is one of the B-complex vitamins called choline, and it is a particular enemy of fat and cholesterol. Curiously, serum choline varies with the season of the year. We are not really sure why, but it is lower in the summer than in the winter. Some researchers believe that it is regulated by ultraviolet light, so that gives us some possibility of controlling it in the future.

The problem of "tired blood" has been well advertised to people who might suffer from iron deficiency. Iron is important in avoiding anemia and a tired feeling. It enables blood to carry the necessary oxygen for normal activity, and it is also an essential part of a crucial enzyme that helps process protein that you have eaten. Normally, serum iron peaks around noon, but with early meals you will have more iron available when you need it to start off full of pep in the morning. It will peak around 7:00 A.M. When you eat only heavy dinners in the evening, the peak of iron energy comes as late as 4:00 or 5:00 P.M., too late in the day to help you much with the day's activities.

Is Thyroid Related to Weight Changes?

Some authorities believe that the thyroid may work to make you fat or make you thin. A low level of thyroid activity delays digestion and, says Broda O. Barnes, M.D., "what is important in weight control is the time food spends in the stomach and intestinal tract." Also involved is a low rate of burning up calories, so that is double trouble! Low thyroid activity is sometimes an explanation for being overweight; Dr. Barnes takes the extreme position of estimating that as many as four people in ten may have a deficient thyroid.

Dr. Barnes also says that "thyroid function decreases with age," so that added years may mean added pounds unless we cut down on calories as we get older (as recommended by the National Academy of Sciences).

One curiosity is that, according to Dr. Barnes again, "a diet high in protein requires additional thyroid." We may be getting to the point when physicians will be recommending more protein for a person with too high a level of thyroid and less protein for those with low thyroid. Perhaps some are already doing that.

The other side of the picture is the attempt by doctors to moderate weight by administering thyroid hormone. Some believe this helps burn up calories. That is, however, a controversial matter that has been carefully reviewed by George A. Bray, Professor of Medicine and Director of the Clinical Research Center at Harbor General Hospital, U.C.L.A. campus at Torrance, California. He writes that "the consensus had gradually evolved that thyroid medication had little to offer," but the issue has been revived since 1963, with more recent studies which again raise the question. It will surely not be resolved here, but Dr. Bray goes on to state that "it is clear that thyroid hormones induce a number of changes in obese patients which will tend to enhance their weight loss." There are, however, undesirable side effects, such as the loss of lean body muscle and consequent loss of nutritionally more important nitrogen. Of more concern are the possible effects on the functioning of the heart.

Dr. Bray concludes that "There is thus no convincing evidence that thyroid hormone produces a more significant and sustained weight loss than carefully administered management using diet as the sole modality of treatment."

It seems that thyroid activity may be related to obesity, at least in some cases, and that this can be affected by diet, and by the timing of the diet.

We do know that low thyroid is associated with weakness and fatigue, headaches, skin problems, repeated infections, menstrual disturbances, loss of memory and ability to concentrate (both are signs of aging), and general depression. Also implicated are high cholesterol and blood pressure. People with low thyroid tend to feel cold and have a persistently low temperature, less than 97.8° F. They perspire less than other people and—most importantly from our point of view—they tend to gain weight, if only by retention of water in the body cells.

High thyroid levels are much less common and are associated with high temperature, sweating, nervous movement and loss of weight. All this is for physicians to look into and diagnose. What concerns us is the fact that thyroid level is affected by the kind of food you eat and when you eat it.

Governing the thyroid level is the hormone TSH (thyroid stimulating hormone). It is high during the night from about 10:00 P.M. to 2:00 A.M. One of the results is an increased flow of a thyroid hormone (thyroxine) that stimulates the appetite. That may be one of the reasons you are tempted to raid the refrigerator at night! Be on guard!

Rhythms and the Growth Hormone

Another hormone has a lot to do with healthy growth and at the same time counteracts the fattening effect of insulin. Appropriately, it is called the growth hormone. It is important to all of us in maintaining healthy bodies, but it is absolutely essential for the healthy growth of a child. This hormone is present in all parts of the body, and it peaks in circulation within a few hours of your going to sleep. The deeper you sleep the more readily it will flow. If you delay sleep you delay the flow of the hormone. Eating meals early in the day brings on the hormone earlier, to peak around 8:00 P.M. Late meals shift much of the flow late into the night and early morning, around 4:00 A.M.

Bad news again for people who are overly plump: those excess pounds reduce the effectiveness of the hormone and reduce the level of it. That's double trouble again. The fatter you are, the less this hormone can help you fight fat. We have some good news, though. If you get out and exercise you can bolster the flow of the hormone. It is not just that you will lose pounds with steady, regular exercise. You will get more deep sleep and more growth hormone to help fight fat and build the proper body tissue.

One indicator of proper protein digestion is a byproduct in the blood called BUN (blood urea nitrogen). The BUN rhythm indicates when the protein you have eaten is being used by your body. When meals are eaten early, the peak occurs before 4:00 P.M., while late meals cause a delay of 12 hours, until the middle of the night.

Significantly, the Halbergs announced at an international nutrition conference that "by manipulating mealtimes for those on a quantitatively usual caloric intake, the timing of circadian rhythms can be changed. Thus, utilization of both food and medications probably will be amenable to optimization."

Getting in Tune with Our Rhythms

Perhaps the day will come when we will all optimize our natural rhythms by paying more attention to what we eat and when we eat, by paying more attention to when we can work best and when we should rest or relax. Gradually, by scientific experiments, we are coming to learn how this can be done.

There could soon come a time when athletes will negotiate the hour of their sports events and will prep themselves by planning their diet to be in top winning form at the crucial hour. Businessmen and diplomats may schedule their big decisions for certain hours when their judgment is best. Doctors can plan their activities for when the patient is strongest, his resistance at a peak, or the drugs more effective. For many scheduled operations, this would *not* be impractical. I am aware that patients' rhythms may vary. But the individual's rhythms may be analyzed, or at least verified. The individual's rhythms may also be altered deliberately.

Meanwhile, we can all benefit by planning our eating more carefully. The key lies in limiting any excess food, and in eating most of the day's rations early, well before nighttime. Again, we should eat breakfast like a king, lunch like a prince, and dinner like a pauper. Along with balanced nutrition and sensible exercise, that is the heart of the Body Clock Diet.

10

THE BODY CLOCK DIET

There is plenty of leeway for personal food preferences—or dislikes—when you plan your own diet menu for the
Body Clock Diet. You can even make a place for special favor-
ites, even if they are fattening, as long as you strictly limit the
amounts and be careful about WHEN you eat them.

Any gastronome, or tea- or wine-taster, can tell you that it is
the first small taste that gives you most of the pleasure. It is your
mouth and nose that do the tasting, not your stomach. Relish the
small morsel and enjoy it all the more.

Most people can go on eating the same foods they are eating
now and lose weight if they will just eat them earlier in the day.
Mostly, though, we eat far too much for our own good. Just about
everyone is somewhat overweight because most people eat far
more than their bodies need and eat the wrong kinds of food at
the wrong times.

If you are already following a diet plan, you can still make your
own body clock work for you by shifting your meals to an earlier
hour. You will lose even more weight! So even if your present
diet is working well you can make it more effective and gain
an advantage that will allow you some extra treats without
gaining a pound.

Now let's look again at what most of us are doing with our
meals, besides eating far too much. We are eating three-quarters

123

of our day's calories in the evening, when we need them least. And we are starving ourselves at breakfast. In perhaps half of all American families, at least one person is skipping breakfast completely. In three-quarters of the families, eating breakfast is no longer done together, so it is usually a grab-something-on-the-run affair. Also, one person in five skips lunch, though few of us fail to eat dinner, and even overeat at dinner. That is what has to change if we are to stay healthy and keep a trim figure

The idea is to eat well, even eat more meals during the day (not night!). Never skip a meal unless you are deliberately fasting.

Set an Example for Your Family

Wherever possible, it would be best if the family could reinstate the old tradition of eating together. Certainly with young children, that is quite possible, to ensure a good hearty meal to start the day. If breakfast together is not possible, food should be handy so that each person can get a full breakfast without a lot of fuss. I also recommend a midmorning snack, a solid lunch, a midafternoon snack, and a very light dinner. It may take a couple of weeks to adapt to it, but it would help a lot if as many as three-quarters of your calories were consumed through the day, with only 25 to 30 percent of your calories saved for the evening meal. And no late-night snacks!

Start by taking larger breakfasts and adequate lunches. You will find that you are less hungry at night. Hard to believe, perhaps, but true. You will find it easier to cut down on dinner when you have eaten enough early in the day.

That does not mean that dinner has to be less of a family affair. It is still best to eat together, to talk, to feel each other's presence, to have all the warmth of company, friendship and love at the dinner table. But care and quality, not quantity, are the keystones to loving preparation of a meal. Challenge your ingenuity in keeping the calories and quantities down.

Most important, though, is to change one's own eating habits.

Whether or not the rest of the family follows suit is ultimately up to them. It is up to us to change our own habits (though of course, it is easier if husband and wife do it together). But if the spouse is going to grouse about this, let it be. And concentrate on your own waistline first. We may not be able to change others much, but we can change ourselves. Your setting an example just might be an inspiration to the others, especially when they see the effect it has on your figure.

The crux of the matter is to take an ample breakfast, an adequate lunch, and a light dinner. Mid-morning and mid-afternoon snacks should be planned, not impromptu, and should rarely exceed 100 to 150 calories.

What to Eat

A limited but balanced diet is recommended by virtually all nutritionists as the best and safest way to control weight. This requires that we know something about the nutritional and caloric value of the basic foods. And it requires that we modify both our attitudes toward eating and our eating behavior.

Sound and balanced diet plans are actually much alike in basic principles, though the foods used may offer a lot of variety. A lot of the good basic ideas have come to be known as the "Prudent Diet," spelled out twenty-five years ago by the late Norman Jolliffe, M.D., who had been Director of the Bureau of Nutrition at New York City's Department of Health.

The food plans were designed not only for weight reduction but also for reduction of coronary problems. In outline, if not in all specifics, they have had the support of eminent experts such as Henry Sebrell, M.D., formerly professor at Columbia Medical School, and Dr. Jean Mayer, formerly professor of nutrition at Harvard University, now president of Tufts University. The nutritional aspects of this diet come, then, with good credentials. It is proven safe and effective even without the added advantages of early timing and supplementary fiber. With few modifications, it amounts to this: For most women (or any adult with a small frame), 1200 calories a day is about right as a basis for losing weight. Most men (or any adult with a large frame) may manage better with 1500 to 1600 calories a day. These are the basic plans, and if the foods are chosen with reasonable care, they provide adequate nutrition for the average person while losing weight. For greater needs, or for maintenance rather than reduction of weight, you can add extra food in specified units of 50 or 100 calories until you find the right level for you. That level might be increased, for example, if you become much more physically active.

Meat such as beef, pork, or lamb, should be limited to no more than 1 pound a week, after bones and all visible fat are removed. This is taken in portions of two to four ounces, according to the menu plan. Once a week it is well to substitute liver, kidneys, or other organ meat in place of a meal of red meat.

Poultry can be served two or more times a week, for a good source of protein with fewer calories and at lower cost. Again, it is best if visible fat is removed.

Seafood should be eaten four to five times a week, with portions planned as two, four, or six ounces. Fish or scallops provide complete protein with few of the nutritional disadvantages of red meat. Shellfish or shrimp are good for one portion of seafood each week. More than that would have disadvantages in terms of cholesterol. Tuna fish should be the kind packed in water, not oil. There is a big difference in the number of calories.

Up to four ounces of hard cheese a week are all right, but only as a substitute for four ounces of red meat. Low-fat cottage cheese is another story, and at least one cup a week is recommended, usually taken in half-cup servings.

You should eat no more than four eggs per week. Eggs have excellent, complete protein, but too many of them might supply too much cholesterol. If you make an omelet, use just two eggs per person.

Milk: Two cups a day of skim milk or buttermilk, or two-thirds cup of non-fat dry milk, or up to one cup of plain, low-fat yogurt (not sweet-flavored) are recommended.

Bread and cereal foods: Eat at least three slices of high-fiber bread a day, and preferably five slices or more. Be sure your bread has at least 5 percent non-nutritive crude fiber; you can't always trust the words "high fiber" on bread labels. An alternative is to use whole-wheat bread (not just wheat bread) and supplementary unprocessed bran, taken at two or more occasions through the day, a tablespoon or two at a time. The bran is readily mixed with other foods, soups, or beverages. Equivalent to two slices of bread is one cup of cooked cereal or one and a half cups of dry cereal (not presweetened).

Fats and oils: Use no more than three teaspoons of vegetable oil (corn, safflower, or soya oil) each day, or the same amount of polyunsaturated margarine. Do not use the oil for frying, but rather for salads and dressing. The margarine is best used on bread, or to add taste to vegetables, potatoes, or rice.

Potatoes or substitute: Once a day, a medium-sized potato, or substitute—sweet potato or yam, one small ear of corn, a half-cup of corn kernels, peas, or green lima beans, or the same amount of rice, spaghetti, macaroni, noodles or grits.

Vegetables should be eaten twice a day, or at least in generous quantities. Most people do not eat enough of them, although they are vitamin rich, often especially in vitamin A. Examples are broccoli, carrots, chicory, collards, escarole, pumpkin, spinach, squash, watercress. Be sure not to use too much water and not to overcook the vegetables. Better yet, use a steamer to preserve the flavor and the vitamins.

Fruit: Eat three fruits a day, preferably fresh, with no added sugar or cream. For variety, they may be taken as juice or mixed in a blender. Once a day it is best to have one fruit high in vitamin C. Good choices are one medium orange (or four ounces of orange juice), half a grapefruit (or four ounces of juice), half a cantaloupe, a cup of strawberries, a tangerine, or eight ounces of tomato juice. You might like to select different combinations of fruits from the following list or combine them to make a fruit cocktail. Be sure, however, to watch the amounts carefully if you do so, and plan on a one-half-cup portion.

127

1 apple, pear, peach, or banana

2–3 apricots, plums, or prunes

¼ pound cherries or grapes

½ cup of natural, unsweetened pineapple

½ honeydew melon

½ cup of berries

½ round slice of watermelon, 1 x 10 inches

2 tablespoons of raisins

½ papaya

1 mango

Certain foods can be eaten freely; they are listed in Exhibit 10–1. Included are many of the leafy vegetables that are filling and nutritious but have a low caloric content. Certain other foods are best avoided, especially at first, to keep the meal plans simple, easy, and nutritionally safe. You should definitely avoid foods fried in oil or butter, and the empty calories in sugared foods. You hardly ever need them. Some foods may be too high in salt, saturated fats, or cholesterol, or they may contain too many calories for your needs. They are listed in Exhibit 10–2. I advise against most dietetic foods because they are usually overpriced. Many are even deceptive in that they still contain too many calories and unhealthful additives and not enough of the needed nutrients.

A basic meal plan for 1200 calories a day is shown in Exhibit 10–3. If you find that you are losing weight too rapidly, or if you are on a regimen of more calories, you can plan on supplements that are listed in Exhibit 10–4. For best control, stay with the basic number of calories you have decided upon, until your weight is clearly where you want it. The day's meal plan should be set up in advance and always monitored with caution.

In my experience, a dietary scale is a necessity. This will ensure that you stay carefully within the allotments. Preferably get one that reads in grams as well as ounces, since many food labels have already converted to the metric system. Cup and spoon measures should also be handy and be used daily, leaving little or nothing to judgment. It is the only way of being objective.

A Suggested Seven-Day Menu

Let's look more closely at a basic model for the week's menu, set at approximately 1200 calories a day. This is arranged with about 30 percent of the day's rations in the evening and with breakfast having about the same amount of food as lunch. Experience suggests that this is the best way to work one's way into more generous breakfasts and lighter dinners. The body system adjusts readily and, in time, breakfasts can be made more substantial than the lunches.

Most of the foods suggested are quite familiar and are easily prepared without a lot of fuss. As you become accustomed to larger breakfasts, then you can try for greater variety and more elaborate dishes. To begin though, simplicity is best. We do need to spell out the specifics of the foods listed in our basic seven-day menu.

Juice for breakfast is always a good way of taking one of your thrice-daily fruits. A half cup, or four ounces, is a good measure. Freshly prepared juice is best, with the natural pulp included. It is well to vary the juice from time to time during the week: orange or apple, pineapple or pear, perhaps tomato juice for a change, or your own blend of papaya, mango or peach, processed in a blender. If you buy the juice in a can, make sure it has not been sweetened.

Cereal: Most people are used to the typical commercial brands —corn flakes, bran flakes, rice puffs or crisps—and half a cup of that is sufficient, or one shredded wheat biscuit. Do not use any presweetened cereal; it is cheaper to add your own sugar and much better yet to use no sugar at all.

Sweetness is best provided by adding your own fresh breakfast fruit to the cereal. Natural fruit sugar is much better for you than table sugar, or sucrose. Raisins are also a good sweetener and count only 30 calories for a measured tablespoon. Also, if

129

THE EFFECTS OF THE BODY CLOCK

Exhibit 10–1. Have as much as you like of these foods and beverages.

Alfalfa sprouts
Asparagus
Beans, green
Beet greens
Beets, red
Bouillon
Broccoli
Brussels sprouts
Cabbage
Calorie-free soft drinks
Capers
Cauliflower
Celery
Chard
Chicory greens
Chili pepper
Chinese cabbage
Chives
Cinnamon (no sugar)
Clam juice
Coffee, black
Collard greens
Cranberries (unsweetened)
Cucumber
Curry powder
Dandelion greens
Dill
Dill pickles (not sweet)
Duruka (Fiji asparagus)
Eggplant
Endive
Escarole
Fennel
Gelatin (unsweetened)
Herbs

Kale
Kohlrabi
Lemon
Lemonade (calorie-free)
Lettuce
Lime
Mung bean sprouts
Mushrooms
Nutmeg
Okra
Onion
Parsley
Pepper, black
Pepper, green or red
Pickles, unsweetened
Pimiento
Radishes
Rhubarb (unsweetened)
Romaine
Sauerkraut
Scallions
Snap beans
Soda water
Soybean sprouts
Spices
Spinach
Summer squash
Taro leaves
Tea, plain
Tomatoes
Truffles
Turnip greens
Vinegar
Water
Watercress

Exhibit 10–2. Have these foods hardly ever, or never, until you reach your desired weight. After you have reached your desired weight, nothing is totally forbidden, but these foods do not help the dieter. If you are losing weight too rapidly, you may want to use small portions of those marked with an asterisk; the others are high in saturated fat, sugar or salt and you are better off without them.

Alcoholic beverages*
Avocado*
Bacon
Beans & pork
Beer*
Biscuits*
Brownies
Butter
Cake
Candy
Canned meats
Carob*
Cereal, presweetened
Chewing gum, unless calorie-
    free
Chili con carne
Chocolate
Cinnamon sugar
Cookies
Corned beef
Corn chips
Corn syrup
Crackers*
Cream
Cream cheese
Cream powder (non-dairy
    creamer)
Cream sauce
Custard
Danish pastry
Dietetic foods
Doughnuts
French fries
Fried chicken
Fried foods, of any sort
Fruit canned in syrup
Fruit juice, sweetened
Hamburger bun*
Hollandaise sauce

Honey
Hot dog
Ice cream
Ice cream soda
Ice milk
Jam
Jelly
Ketchup
Maple syrup
Mayonnaise
Muffins*
Non-dairy creamer
Olives
Olive oil
Pancakes*
Pastrami
Pastry
Popcorn*
Potato chips
Potato salad
Pretzels
Processed meats
Puddings
Salad dressings, bottled
Salami
Salted nuts
Sausage
Soda crackers*
Soft drinks, unless calorie-free
Steak, marbled
Sugar
Sweet pickles
Syrup, any kind
Tartar sauce
Waffles*
Whipped cream
White sauce
Whole milk

you simply chew the cereal slowly, the enzymes in your mouth will convert some of the starch to glucose, and replace the need for any added sugar.

Fortified cereals are more concentrated sources of nutrition than the traditional flakes, and there are several good brands of high-protein cereals on the market. Use only one-quarter to one-third of a cup of these. One of the best ideas, and my favorite, is toasted wheat germ (quarter cup), with two tablespoons of unprocessed bran flakes. Add a half dozen plain, unsalted almonds to the cereal for additional protein, lively flavor, and an agreeable way of packing in more morning energy.

Add no more than one-half cup of skim milk. Or mix the cereal with one-half cup of low-fat yogurt for an even more nutritious breakfast. That is an interesting switch, especially useful for people who just do not like milk or are allergic to it.

Yogurt should equal half a cup of the plain low-fat kind, with no added flavorings, because all the commercial flavorings are sugar-based. Your own flavoring may be added by way of your fresh morning fruit, sliced and added to the yogurt. My passion is for berries in the yogurt—a glorious cup of fresh strawberries in season, with half a cup of low-fat yogurt.

Skim milk is the only milk adults ever need. It may be used on the cereal and in the tea or coffee. Use no sugar, only artificial sweeteners if you feel the need. Surprisingly, it is not hard to wean oneself away from a heavy dependence on sweetness. Most of us just never thought about it or really tried to do without it for several days in a row.

Cottage cheese is a good staple that mixes well with tuna, shrimp, clams, or any fish, meat or poultry that is served cold. Use the low-fat cottage cheese (1 percent milkfat), with no added salt. Most people prefer the cream style to the dry curd variety. It supplies only 90 calories per half-cup serving and provides 30 percent of the day's protein needs. Chopped scallions or chives add color and flavor.

Bread: Best is the high-fiber bread, which some of us like best toasted. When margarine is on the menu, keep it to one-half

Exhibit 10–3. A suggested seven-day menu for 1200 calories a day.

	MONDAY	TUESDAY	WEDNESDAY	THURSDAY	FRIDAY	SATURDAY	SUNDAY
Breakfast	Juice Cereal Milk Toast, 2 slices Margarine Fruit Tea/Coffee	Juice Ham Carrots Bread, 1 slice Tea/Coffee	Juice Flounder Bread, 2 slices Margarine Yogurt Fruit Tea/Coffee	Chicken Milk Bread, 2 slices Fruit Tea/Coffee	Juice Haddock Bread, 2 slices Margarine Yogurt Fruit Tea/Coffee	Juice ½ cantaloupe Cereal Milk Nuts Toast, 1 slice Margarine Tea/Coffee	Juice Poached eggs (2) Toast, 2 slices Milk Fruit salad Tea/Coffee
Lunch	Tunafish Cottage cheese Vegetable Lentils Milk	Shrimp Rice Vegetable Bread, 2 slices Milk	Chicken Potato Vegetable Bread, 1 slice Milk	Ground beef Vegetable Bread, 1 slice Milk	Turkey Rice Vegetable Bread, 1 slice Milk	Scallops Corn Vegetable Bread Milk	Roast beef Potato Vegetable Milk
Dinner	Boullion Chicken sandwich Salad Fruit Tea/Coffee	Chowder Flounder Raw vegetable salad Bread, 1 slice Fruit Tea/Coffee	Vegetable juice Omelet Bread, 1 slice Salad Fruit Tea/Coffee	Tunafish Cottage cheese Raw vegetable salad Bread, 1 slice Tea/Coffee	Turkey salad Asparagus Bread, 1 slice Fruit Tea/Coffee	Salmon loaf Vegetable Salad Bread, 1 slice Fruit Tea/Coffee	Grilled cheese sandwich Salad Fruit Tea/Coffee

teaspoon for each slice. More margarine than that does not give more flavor. Many people have found that low-fat yogurt goes well as a spread, saving the margarine for flavoring their daily vegetables, potato or rice.

Morning meat, fish or chicken should be a full serving of four ounces (six ounces for the 1500-calorie regimen), grilled, baked or boiled, but never fried unless you do so in a nonstick pan, without cooking oil. Another "legal" alternative for frying is to use a nonstick pan-spray that should add no more than one calorie per serving.

Bone and all visible fat should be removed before weighing. Many people find it helpful to precook meats in the evening for use the next morning. Then they may be eaten cold or heated quickly if you are rushed when you get up. Luncheon portions are the same size as breakfast portions, but dinner portions are reduced to two ounces on the basic diet.

Ground beef should be the leanest available to you. This may appear to be more expensive than cheaper hamburger meat, but when you realize that you are just getting a lot of unneeded fat in the cheaper meats, you will choose the best and leanest.

Salmon or tuna loaf may be made without any butter, whatever the traditional cookbooks say. Mix a half cup of high-fiber breadcrumbs for each four-ounce can of salmon or tuna, and mix in an egg. Bake for half an hour at 350° or until golden brown on top. A portion is four ounces at breakfast or lunch, and two ounces for supper. Many people find this easy to eat at breakfast, and it is good hot or cold.

Tea is easier on the body than coffee, and millions of British people around the world will tell you that it is just as effective an eye-opener as coffee is in the morning. You may ease up on caffeine by drinking any one of several types of herb teas now sold in most supermarkets, or by using a decaffeinated brand of coffee. You might prefer to get your morning "lift" with regular coffee and switch to the decaffeinated kind after the first cup. It will be easier on the heart and nerves, and will let you enjoy a more peaceful day.

Lentils appear on our menu although some people are not yet accustomed to eating them. They are an excellent food, easily prepared and with a readily appreciated flavor if you are tasting them for the first time. They may be served hot as a vegetable or cold, in a salad. Just cover the dry beans in water and wait half an hour or until the water is mostly absorbed. Then cook for about ten minutes. Do not overcook, or they will become mushy. One-half cup is the proper amount to take of the cooked lentils.

Rice should be served in half-cup amounts, measured after cooking. "Potato" means a small to medium one, not one of the huge baking potatoes. If you buy the larger types, cut them to weighed portions of three and a half ounces. Home fries and French fries are out; they absorb too much fat. You can get a somewhat similar effect, and just as tasty, if you boil the potatoes lightly, slice them, and put them under a grill, turning them occasionally with a watchful eye so they do not burn. With a little care you can make them golden crisp.

Chicken or tuna sandwiches are to be made with two slices of high-fiber bread. No mayonnaise should be used unless your regimen allows an extra 50-calorie supplement for one tablespoon of imitation mayonnaise. A good substitute is low-fat yogurt, with added chives or onion, and as much lettuce as you like. In the same way, a delicious turkey salad can be adapted by using yogurt instead of mayonnaise.

Make a grilled cheese sandwich for yourself with high-fiber toast. Put a slice of toast with cheese under the broiler for a minute to melt the cheese and then put the second slice of toast on top.

Chowder should not contain potatoes, just clams, clam juice, skim milk or yogurt, and spices to taste.

Supplements for More Energy

Menus for more than 1200 calories a day may be adapted from the same basic pattern. For 1600 calories a day, supplements may be added for the additional 400 calories, always with an eye to keeping the bulk of them to the early meals.

THE EFFECTS OF THE BODY CLOCK

The easiest and best way to add nutrients is to increase the poultry and fish portions of the menu. An additional four ounces will add about 200 calories. Two extra slices of high-fiber bread will bring in another 100 calories, or 150 if you add a half teaspoon each of margarine and preserves.

Especially at first, the best solution is to increase the size of portions already being served, rather than picking over a wide variety of other tempting foods. The more decisions you ponder, the harder it is. However, to get you settled into a routine, I have listed a wide variety of supplements in amounts of approximately 50, 100 and 200 calories in Exhibits 10–4, 10–5 and 10–6. My firm advice, though, is to stay with the sound nutrient basics until you are maintaining your desired weight, and you might then look for more variety.

Exhibit 10–4. Fifty-calorie supplements to modify the basic 1200-calorie menu plan for weight loss.

Supplement	Amount
Almonds	8
Apricots, diced halves	3
Artichokes	1 large
Bread, high-fiber	1 slice
Cashew nuts	5
Chestnuts	5
Chicken liver	1
Clam dip	2 tbsp.
Coconut milk	1 cup
Corn syrup	1 tbsp.
Crabmeat	1/2 cup
Crackers, plain	4
Cream, heavy	1 tbsp.
Cream, light	1 1/2 tbsp.
Cream, whipped	2 tbsp.
Cream cheese	1 tbsp.
Dates	3
Graham crackers	4
Green peas	1/2 cup

THE BODY CLOCK DIET

Supplement	Amount
Half-and-half	2 tbsp.
Jam or jelly	1 tbsp.
Ketchup	3 tbsp.
Imitation bacon	2 tbsp.
Imitation mayonnaise	1 tbsp.
Maple syrup	1 tbsp.
Marshmallows	2
Olives	5
Peanuts	10
Pecans	5
Pistachio nuts	15
Plums, fresh	2
Popcorn, popped	½ cup
Potato chips	5
Pretzel sticks, thin	10
Raisins	2 tbsp.
Relish	2 tbsp.
Shortbread cookie	1
Soda crackers	2
Sugar	1 tbsp.
Tartar sauce	1 tbsp.
Tomato juice	4 ounces
Vanilla wafers	2
Walnuts	6

Exhibit 10–5. One-hundred calorie supplements to modify the basic 1200-calorie menu plan for weight loss. (One glass is 8 oz).

Supplement	Amount
Ale	1 glass
Almonds	15
Apple juice, unsweetened	1 cup
Applesauce, unsweetened	1 cup
Bacon	2 strips
Banana	1 medium
Beer	1 glass
Berries	1 cup
Biscuit, 2-inch diameter	1
Brownie	1 small

Supplement	Amount
Butter	1 tbsp.
Cantaloupe	one-half medium
Carbonated soft drink	1 glass
Cheese, Camembert	1 ounce
Cheese, cheddar	1 ounce
Cherries, fresh	25
Chicken, drumstick	1
Chocolate mint	1
Chowder, Manhattan	1 cup
Clams	12
Cocoa	1 cup with 3 ounces milk, 3 ounces water
Cola	1 glass
Cole slaw	1 cup
Cookies, chocolate chip	2
Corn flakes	1 cup
Cottage cheese, low fat	$1/2$ cup
Crabmeat	1 cup
Cream, heavy	2 tbsp.
Cream, whipped topping	$2/3$ cup
Dates	5
Doughnut	1 small
Egg noodles, cooked	$1/2$ cup
Farina, cooked	1 cup
Gelatin, flavored	$2/3$ cup
Gin	$1 1/2$ ounces
Grape juice	4 ounces
Grape nuts	$1/4$ cup
Grapefruit	1
Grapes, seedless	1 cup
Hard roll	1
Herring, canned	2 ounces
Ice cream	$1/3$ cup
Lentils, cooked	$1/2$ cup
Lima beans	$1/2$ cup
Liquor, 80 proof	$1 1/2$ ounces
Lobster	$3/4$ pound
Macaroon	1
Margarine	1 tbsp.
Mayonnaise	1 tbsp.
Minestrone	1 cup

THE BODY CLOCK DIET

Supplement	Amount
Noodles	1/2 cup
Orange	1 large
Orange juice	1 cup
Oatmeal cookie	1
Oyster soup, creamed	1 cup
Peaches, canned, water pack	1 cup
Peanut butter	1 tbsp.
Pear, fresh	1
Popover	1
Potato	1 medium
Potato chips	9 average size
Prunes	5
Rice, cooked	1/2 cup
Saltines	8
Sardines	1
Shrimp, canned	3 ounces
Soup	
Cream of chicken	1 cup
Tomato	1 cup
Vegetable beef	1 cup
Swiss cheese	1 ounce
Table wine	3 1/2 ounces
Tangerines	2
Wheat germ	3 tbsp.
Whisky	1 1/2 ounces

Exhibit 10–6. Two-hundred calorie supplements to modify the basic 1200-calorie menu plan for weight loss.

Supplement	Amount
Avocado	one-half medium
Bacon	4 strips
Bagel, with 1 tbsp. margarine	1
Beef	4 ounces
Beef stew	1 cup
Beef patty	4 ounces
Bread, each slice with 1 tsp. margarine	
and 1 tsp. jam	2 slices
Chicken	4 ounces
Corned beef hash	2/3 cup

Supplement	Amount
Custard pudding	$2/3$ cup
Eel	4 ounces
Fish	4 ounces
Ice milk	1 cup
Lima beans	1 cup
Lamb chop, rib or shoulder	1
Macaroni, cooked	1 cup
Margarine	1 ounce (2 tbsp.)
Meat	4 ounces
Noodles	1 cup
Pancakes	3 small
Peas, dried, cooked	$2/3$ cup
Pizza	1 slice
Pork chop, loin	1
Pork sausages	2 links (3″ x $1/2$″)
Potato, whipped, with 1 tbsp. margarine	$3/4$ cup
Potato	1 large
Rice, cooked	$3/4$ cup
Sardines	2
Scallops	6
Spaghetti, cooked	1 cup
Tunafish, water-packed	$3/4$ cup
Turkey	4 ounces
Waffle	1
Wheat germ	$1/2$ cup

Besides more poultry, fish or bread, you can increase your calories with low-fat cottage cheese, rice, potatoes, lentils, or fruit. Other foods are listed in case you have a particular favorite and you choose to add that. Remember though, the supplement lists contain some foods and beverages (like liquor), that do not give you much except calories with a flavor.

The keystone of success, we find, is to keep the menu plan simple and routine, so you are not burdened each meal, each day, by a lot of difficult decisions about what to eat and what not to eat. Simplicity of the menu and advance planning once a week is the answer.

Each meal or snack must be treated with respect, caution and concentration—nothing casual, nothing careless, always carefully weighing and checking until you know the routine by heart and there is little danger of deviation. Do not torture yourself with a hundred little decisions—and if in doubt, do not eat what you are thinking about.

If you feel you are going to crash, put it off until the next breakfast, when you can have plenty to eat anyway, more than your fill, because nature controls your overeating then, and copes better with overindulgence.

Finally, be careful you do not lose too much weight too fast, or continue to lose after you have reached your desired goal. A weekly weighing is a good idea to monitor your own progress. Do it at the same time of the day each week because weight varies in a periodic cycle each day.

After you have achieved your goal, add no more than 50 calories a day for a week, to find your maintenance level. If you are still losing weight, add another 50 calories a day during the next week, and so on, till you find the exact level of energy intake that will keep you safely trim at the weight you want.

How to Eat Breakfast When You Don't Feel Like It

It may be a long way off but the day could come when you have steak, potato and vegetables for breakfast. That's what we had when I was a schoolboy back in Australia. It was often served topped with eggs and preceded by porridge. Even for adults Down Under, such generous breakfasts are traditionally part of any bed-and-board living arrangement, whether it be in city or country. It is good to start the day with a hearty meal.

A couple of poached eggs, toast, juice and coffee are traditional, even in the United States. Add a piece of fruit, some milk and cereal and you have half a day's calories for a diet of 1200 calories a day. Six hundred calories may be too much for you in the morning, but you should aim for at least 420 calories at that first meal of the day, to equal 35 percent of the day's rations.

In the morning, fish and poultry usually go down easier than red meat, and are better for you. Along with juice or fruit, and a cereal with milk, you might put away three or four ounces of fish or poultry. But use the grill or broiler. You should not fry in fat at all, at any time. Doing most of the cooking the night before can mean that you have more time in the morning to enjoy your meal.

If you are not used to meat or eggs in the morning, you can load in the calories with fruit, yogurt and cereal, supplemented with unsalted almonds, raisins and skim milk. For the cereal I recommend wheat germ rather than the commercial brands, and certainly not the presweetened brands. A number of the commercial concentrates are all right.

I and many people who follow this diet put together our own concoction of cereal with different proportions according to personal taste. Sometimes I put a poached egg on top and eat the fruit separately. It can always help to put in up to two tablespoons of unprocessed bran flakes. That is a good 10 percent fiber, and you will want to spread your fiber intake throughout the day, divided among your meals or snacks. Take the fiber in small amounts at first, perhaps a tablespoon at a time until your system adapts to the healthier regimen. Some very sensitive people may have to start with only a teaspoon at a time, but the amount should be increased as the body adapts.

Some People Can't Eat Breakfast at All

Some people, and you may be one of them, simply can't eat breakfast at all. Coffee or tea and that's it. They do not feel like food then, and the idea is even repulsive. I have heard that a thousand times. Almost a thousand times I have also found that those people can learn to down a lot of calories with good nutrition, and enjoy it, if they will follow some easy advice on how to choose their foods.

One secret is to drink your breakfast. A high-protein drink can pack enough energy and nutrients to keep you going for hours. One of my favorite recipes is Beverly and Vidal Sassoon's Vitality Drink that loads 230 calories per glass. Their recipe is as good as you will find, and serves two people. Use your blender and, if you like, a little imagination to vary the ingredients.

2 tablespoons powdered protein
1 tablespoon granular lecithin
1 large banana
1 raw egg (optional)
2 cups low-fat or skim milk

You can readily double the amount of powdered protein and skip the lecithin, which has not been proved to have all the value claimed for it by enthusiasts.

If you cannot drink milk, use low-fat yogurt instead. Fruit juice, low-fat yogurt or skim milk, and protein powder are all good bases for a liquid breakfast. Fruit of almost any sort blends in well, as does a raw or boiled egg. I add two tablespoons of unprocessed bran flakes for additional B vitamins and iron. Wheat germ is a healthy addition too, giving you 110 calories per quarter-cup serving. Wheat germ, nuts, raisins, all mix well to give ample energy in a liquid or semi-liquid breakfast.

One caution: Some of the commercial high-protein breakfast products are sugar-based or flavored with sugars, whether they are protein powders, liquids, so-called nutrition bars or "instant" breakfasts. Often, sugar is 40 to 70 percent of the ingredients. Fat may be 25 to 30 percent of the ingredients, mostly saturated fats, according to *Consumer Reports*. My advice is to avoid them unless they are sugar-free and low in saturated fats. Read the labels. It is the only way to be sure. And if you do use the sugar-based products, tote a toothbrush for a good cleaning after such a snack or meal in order to avoid problems with your teeth later on.

Try the liquid breakfast, if only once or twice, to convince yourself that it goes down easily, even if you hate the thought of breakfast. Come mid-morning, you will notice the difference in how you feel. It is hard to describe. You just feel better, more alive, more alert and efficient. This becomes obvious once you start asking yourself how you feel, noticing your own energy level and assessing the change that has occurred. As I have said before, most of us are oblivious to how we feel and do not realize that we could feel a lot better if we energized our day with a good breakfast.

There is another difficulty often mentioned in connection with a big breakfast. You are hurried in the morning. There is no time for breakfast and you are anxious to get the kids packed off to school and get ready for work yourself. Every five minutes of additional sleep seems precious.

Of course it helps to plan on getting up a bit earlier and going to bed a bit earlier. Have the food precooked, ready and accessible in the proper portions. It does not take much time to whip up a protein drink, make some toast and coffee and down a piece of fruit. And whatever time it takes is worth it in the way you will feel later.

Breakfast Is the Most Important Meal of the Day

Breakfast is definitely the most important meal of the day. It is staggering to see an Iowa study reporting that 50 to 70 percent of students go to school without breakfast. And there is a Massachusetts study showing that 95 percent of the youngsters go to school there without an adequate breakfast. A few years ago, the American Medical Association Council on Foods and Nutrition concluded that an adequate breakfast is eaten in only 20 percent of American households.

I lived for many years in the South Sea Islands, in Fiji, and was interested in what the islanders have to teach us in the art of living with a minimum of unnecessary stress. One of their secrets is revealed by the fact that the one meal that merits a special name is breakfast, called "katalau." No one would dream of starting the day without breakfast, and heavy, late-night dinners are unknown. Closer to nature and to the needs and feelings of their bodies, Fijians have intuitively learned traditions that make nutritional sense.

We too may learn to adapt our eating habits to live in accord with our biological nature. Even if we turn away from solid

144

food in the morning hours, we can begin the re-education process by drinking the first meal of the day. Then we can find our way back to eating the calorie-rich and more traditional foods such as eggs, toast and cereal.

In all my experience, I have never known a person who could not take soft foods or liquids in the morning and feel the better for it. Those who persistently said they could not do it, I have always felt, never gave it a fair try. Perhaps, for whatever reason, they really had not reached a full commitment to controlling their weight, to freeing themselves of using food as an emotional crutch in the late hours of the night, or of succumbing to social pressure to eat heavily in the evening, when the body needs little nourishment. One has to learn to say no to evening indulgence, and the easiest way to manage that is to have eaten a generous breakfast in the morning.

The simple fact is that a hearty breakfast diminishes any later urges to gorge at the wrong time. I am convinced, and experience supports this, that if you will try carefully for two weeks to eat generous breakfasts, you will never go back to skipping that meal and you will have proved to yourself how much better you feel. You will marvel at how you functioned for so long without realizing this. No words I can say will convince you as well as your own experience by doing it. Try it and see the difference. Give it a fair try, not just a day or two, but a full two weeks. You will never turn back to your old self-destructive eating habits. You will feel like a new person.

Part Four
THE EFFECTS OF DIETARY FIBER

11

FIBER CAN HELP REGULATE YOUR BODY

Irregularity is a serious problem for millions of people in the United States and all over the world who eat a modern diet. So common is the problem among the elderly that many, if not most, younger people can expect to find themselves bound up with the problem, unless they personally decide to do something about it. Meanwhile, almost everyone has experienced the problem at some time. A shame, because it is almost all really quite unnecessary.

Constipation is no problem with rural people in the less developed countries. When I lived in the South Sea Islands and worked closely with herbal medicine there, I never heard the complaint except in the towns where people had adopted modern English or French foods. The same observation has emerged from the work of British scientists in Africa. It never occurred to me why this was so until these scientists discovered how much our Western diet has in recent decades moved away from healthy foods, and they recognized the importance of this. As more people have managed to earn better incomes, they have changed their eating habits in extremely dangerous ways.

According to *Consumer Reports,* over 700 laxative products are sold in the United States, and almost all of them should be unnecessary. Except for very restricted and uncommon cases, the

149

problem can be solved by carefully choosing what you eat and when you eat it, as well as by easing up on worry and anxiety and by taking appropriate exercise. Says the usually reliable *Consumer Reports* in their book *The Medicine Show,* "constipation caused by organic disease is not common. In general, if constipation has been present for years, the likelihood is that it is not due to serious disease."

Laxatives Cause Constipation

Chronic use of laxatives, in fact, is one of the main causes of chronic constipation and, says *Consumer Reports,* "If you think you have chronic constipation, the first thing to do is to stop taking laxatives. Many people who have done so at the insistence of a doctor have been surprised to find that, after a few days or a week, the bowels begin to move effectively again." Temporary constipation usually cures itself, and temporary irregularity need not be cause for concern or for the use of laxatives, especially in the case of children.

The Natural Way to Regularity

The natural way to regularity is through the inclusion of natural fiber in the diet, distributed among the various meals or snacks of the day.

A healthy, natural diet might not require supplements of fiber, but few people in the United States ordinarily eat enough fruit, vegetables or whole-grain products. We do need deliberately to choose such foods for the fiber content as well as for the other nutrients.

This is easier said than done. Most processed foods have the fiber removed, or have little fiber to begin with, and practically all of us are eating more of our foods in processed and prepared form. What then should we do to see that we get enough fiber?

The best answer is still through care in trying to select a balanced diet of foods that you do enjoy, with concentration on fruits, vegetables and cereals, rather than sweets, red meats and other high-calorie, low-fiber foods. Specific foods recommended for fiber content are wheat bran and carrots and other root vegetables, especially when they are not overcooked. For this purpose, plain wheat bran is better than the more expensive, prepackaged, breakfast bran cereals. Whole-grain breads can be used regularly, but there is much more fiber in commercial high-fiber bread now on the market, which has as much as 7.5 percent fiber by weight.

When you eat enough fiber, the changes in your system are conspicuous and you will notice them right away. Your stool will be soft and will pass easily, with no straining. It will be practically odor-free and more bulky and frequent. You may not notice it yourself but food in your system will be passed through within the day, not prolonged in transit for days as it is when there is too little fiber.

The ideal is to have varied sources of fiber because there are many different kinds of fiber, each with somewhat different effects on the digestive system. Contrary to popular opinion, scientists do not yet know much about what sorts of fiber are in our different foods, and their is still no good way of measuring the types and amounts of each kind or component of dietary fiber in each food.

Published estimates have almost all been based on "crude fiber," measured by one particular method that fails to take into account much of the dietary fiber. The really effective dietary fiber is almost always more, sometimes very much more, than indicated by the crude fiber estimates.

What Exactly Is "Fiber"?

The definition and measurement of fiber content of food is something that has confused much of the writing on this subject. Fiber is actually composed of several basic substances. Cellulose is a complex carbohydrate that gives fiber a threadlike, fibrous appearance when it is looked at closely. But measures of crude fiber omit up to half the cellulose. Hemicellulose is another, related compound in fiber, though it is less fibrous than cellulose. With lignin, it serves to make the plant cell wall tough.

But 80 percent of the hemicellulose may be omitted in measures of crude fiber. Lignin itself, though not a carbohydrate, is still another ingredient in dietary fiber. It gives plasticity as well as the woody characteristic, but most of that ingredient is missed in measures of crude fiber, though it can have dietary significance. Another component of fiber is pectin, especially present in fruit; it serves to absorb water and thus soften the stool.

The word "roughage" does not tell us much, except as a vague conversational term for fiber. G. A. Spiller, one of the leading authorities in this area, suggests the term "plantix" (abbreviated as PX), from "plant and matrix," to include all the pectins, gums and mucilage, as well as cellulose, hemicellulose and lignin that make up fiber.

How to Add Fiber to Your Diet

We need not bother much with exact definitions of "fiber" until the U.S. Department of Agriculture measures all our foods with whatever new definition and measuring technique they choose. But we should immediately begin ensuring that we get enough, well, let us call it "dietary fiber." We know enough about how to do that to plan a balanced diet that includes enough fiber of different kinds for our bodies' needs. We should eat plenty of vegetables, fruit, and cereal grains, and we should also include either unrefined bran or certain processed foods, such as bread that contains powdered cellulose.

Fruits and vegetables are generously included in our Body Clock Diet Plan, but it is well to supplement them with at least a small amount of bran. Two tablespoons (six teaspoons) of bran a day is not too much for most people, and all the better if that is distributed through the meals or snacks three times a day, with two teaspoons each time. Go gently at first, perhaps just two teaspoons a day, until your system adjusts to the changes. This may cause a little flatulence during the first week or two, but it is mild and not really disturbing. The bacterial inhabitants of your intestinal tract are changing over and adapting for the better. In rare cases, it may take more than a month to adjust to this.

The simplest fiber to buy is the unrefined bran in health food stores, but note that it comes in several sizes of flake, several price levels and in several brands. You will have to experiment to find what is best for you. Hopefully, more supermarkets will carry the product in the future.

Plain bran may be added to almost any other food: gravies, sandwich spreads, soups or sauces, baked in pies or even cakes, added to stew, mixed into a meatloaf or grilled hamburger. It may be sprinkled over breakfast cereal, swirled into a blended beverage, or simply stirred into fruit juice or vegetable juice. The possibilities are almost limitless. It goes well with practically anything.

I even carry a small container of bran when I travel, and use it in restaurants. People hardly notice me sprinkling it on one of my dishes or stirring it into one of my drinks. If they do notice, there is no need to explain anything unless they ask, and I find that a word or two, or a smile, puts them at ease. There is no need for lengthy explanations. They are not that interested, and most of the time no one notices at all.

High-fiber bread is one pleasant and easy way to integrate fiber into the diet. For this purpose, and for a feeling of fullness that helps in a weight-control program, I recommend five or more slices a day, served at two or more meals or snacks. It helps if the bread is truly high fiber, with at least five percent fiber listed on the label. Some bakeries advertise "high fiber" when the bread actually contains much less than that.

Flavored spreads for the high-fiber bread should be sensible, not butter, jam or peanut butter, unless you are on a maintenance diet, and even then you should measure them all carefully. Sensible choices combine some of these ingredients, blended into a base of moist, low-fat cottage cheese, or low-fat, plain yogurt. For added flavor and variety, you may wish to mix in some tuna flakes, salmon, minced clams, or shrimp. For added flavor with a negligible amount of added calories, add some chives or some minced scallions. Polyunsaturated margarine alone may be spread on sparingly, with as little as half a teaspoon giving ample flavor to a piece of bread or toast; it is the flavor, not so much the fat, that we want to add to the basic cereal product with fiber.

A pause for moderation now: Too much of a good thing is a bad thing. Even too much water can be harmful. Any product can be harmful when taken in excess, and fiber is no exception. However, fiber is in the main a fairly neutral ingredient that does not react much in the body's biochemistry.

There are some indications that excessive plant matrix may bind up available zinc and other minerals that otherwise could be useful to and even necessary for your nutritional health. But the story has not yet been unraveled by scientists. Earlier it was thought that phytate in whole-grain cereals was the key factor in binding zinc—making it unavailable to the body. Research is still being done on that, but as long as you eat a balanced diet and realize that eating anything in excess is dangerous, there is no problem. If it is not the binding-up of zinc, it will be something else. Moderation is the only way. You find the amount of fiber that suits you, and stay with it day in and day out as part of your new life-style of health and weight control.

Long-Range Benefits of Fiber

Aside from helping with daily regularity, fiber is believed to be a preventive for several of the serious illnesses of the modern world. Some scientists make extraordinary claims that might well be true. Other scientists are not completely convinced because a lack of fiber has never been proved to be a direct cause of so many diseases.

Cause and effect may not be proved but the circumstantial evidence is very strongly suggestive. What is clear, and agreed to by virtually all scientists, is that our modern diet is in some ways not nearly as healthy as earlier, more traditional diets of Europe and America, or the modern-day diets among the rural people of less developed parts of the world, such as Africa and some of the South Sea Islands. Those people may be cash poor, but many are rich in good nutrition, in human dignity, and in being closer to finding fulfillment with a pleasant life-style on this earth.

What are the main differences in diet? Well, the amount of fiber in the diet is one of the biggest differences. Some rural Africans eat about 25 grams of crude fiber in their daily diet. In the United States we are more likely to have as little as two grams a day. We eat a huge amount of sugar; they eat very little. We eat a lot of animal fat and, with a few remarkable exceptions, they eat little. They also get a lot more exercise than we do.

The perplexing fact is that rural people in many parts of the world are virtually free of the major ills that are most common to us. Almost all scientists agree that this must be due to differences in diet, partly because when Africans or Pacific Islanders adopt our diet they fall heir to our serious sicknesses, sickness that was not with us in earlier years when we ate much less sugar or red meat and much more whole-grain and root crops or other vegetables. It is more than a fair guess that the long-range effect of a lack of fiber in the diet is deadly.

The conclusion is inevitable: If we want to save our own lives, we must stop killing ourselves with too much food of the wrong sort and return to the generous use of dietary fiber, in whatever form we choose to eat it.

You do not have to return to a nineteenth-century rural diet. That is hardly possible, anyway. But fiber is, I believe, essential to the regulation of your own body rhythms. If you integrate it properly with everyday diet, you will find that it does help regularize your digestion, in accord with your own body processes. It could even save your life.

It is well to look, if only briefly, at those dietary diseases that maim and kill us, to take this message seriously. Infectious diseases have been mostly controlled or conquered by medical scientists. But we ourselves are the only ones who can change our own dietary patterns and conquer or control these dietary diseases. All doctors can do is try to repair some of the damage done.

"It should be emphasized," says Dr. D. M. Hegsted, Professor of Nutrition at Harvard School of Public Health, "that this diet which affluent people generally consume is everywhere associated with a similar disease pattern—high rates of ischemic heart disease, certain forms of cancer, diabetes, and obesity. These are the major causes of death and disability in the United States." He goes on to stress that "these diseases have a complex etiology. It is not correct, strictly speaking, to say that they are caused by malnutrition but rather that an inappropriate diet contributes to their causation. Our genetic makeup contributes— not all people are equally susceptible. Yet those who are genetically susceptible, most of us, are those who would profit most from an appropriate diet."

To Keep a Healthy Heart

The deadly diseases associated with a lack of complex carbohydrates (including fiber) are heart disease and cancer of the digestive tract. Heart attacks account for one-third of all deaths in the United States, and again as many people or more suffer a first heart attack and recover for perhaps an additional five to seven years of life on the average. The damage is never overcome in the sense that a disabled part of the heart can never be regenerated. A causative factor is thrombosis, or a blood clot, which often leads to lung failure (pulmonary embolism) as well, and may also underlie problems of phlebitis (which was brought to the attention of the public when former President Nixon suffered from it). Many scientists believe that such diseases are almost entirely dietary in origin.

Cancer of the digestive tract (the colon and the rectum) is the most common form of deadly cancer in the United States, and it is almost exclusively an avoidable dietary disease. Fiber helps to avert it because the fermentation of fiber contributes to the removal of bowel ammonia. Professor Peter Van Soest of Cornell University Division of Nutritional Sciences explains, "Bowel ammonia, a toxin that results from a high-protein diet, has been suggested as a potential carcinogen that may relate to the high incidence of colon cancer in certain societies, including our own."

The particular value of fiber is the fact that bowel movements are more frequent, and wastes do not linger long in the digestive system. Diverticular disease, the formation of blockages and pouches in the intestinal tract that inhibit bowel movement, is related to slow and even painful bowel movements, as well as the accumulation of wastes in the body. These obstructions and pressured segments of the colon are experienced by 40 percent of all Americans over the age of forty, and they are pandemic among those over seventy. It is reassuring that the *British Medical Journal* reported in 1972 experimental work by Dr. N. S. Painter in which 62 out of 70 patients found relief from symptoms of diverticulitis when they ate a diet high in fiber.

The Diet Is Implicated

Little is known about what causes appendicitis, but appendectomy is the most common abdominal operation in the United States, although appendicitis is practically unknown in rural Africa. Again, the diet is implicated when there is a genuine inflammation and the operation is essential.

Varicose veins strike one-tenth of the U.S. population, yet are extremely rare in rural countries where the diet is healthier. Hemorrhoids are a related problem with the same basic cause, but they affect about half of the U.S. population, and again, are unnecessarily brought on or aggravated by the diet that is lacking in natural fiber.

Much of all this has to do with poor circulation and inflammation of the veins, presenting a spectrum of uncomfortable, if not deadly, diseases that cripple the affluent populations of modern society around the world.

The Diet and Diabetes

Poor circulation is characteristic of diabetes, another dietary disease in that any genetic susceptibility may be aggra-

157

vated by improper diet. A high-carbohydrate, low-fat diet is now often basic to treatment as well as prevention. Obesity is dangerous to anyone, but especially so to diabetics. Indications are that dietary fiber can play a significant role in reducing the dangers.

A recent study gave convincing proof of this before the Midwest Conference of the American Dietetic Association in St. Louis, Missouri. Pearl Miranda and David L. Horwitz of the University of Chicago reported that fiber reduced plasma glucose levels of seven out of eight diabetics who ate twenty grams of fiber a day for ten days. The experiment was designed as a cross-over, with each patient experiencing ten days with the added fiber and ten days without.

Particularly exciting from the point of view of body rhythms was that the effect of fiber became more pronounced through the day, as the fiber was consumed, and declined at night so that blood sugar levels were hardly different by early morning.

The significance for diabetics is extraordinary: The diabetic who eats fiber may be able to reduce the amount of insulin needed as medication. According to Victor T. D. H. Major, M.D., the amount of insulin *must* be reduced on the evidence of such a drop in blood sugar.

All this suggests good news for non-diabetics, too. If blood sugar levels are lowered by fiber, then less fat-forming insulin may be generated by the body when high levels of fiber are added to the diet.

In this University of Chicago experiment with diabetes mellitus, most of the fiber (sixteen of the twenty grams) was provided in the form of high-fiber bread that contained as much as 7 percent dietary fiber. It was the same kind of bread that was used in the weight-loss experiments I worked with over a period of several years.

Can Fiber Help Control Weight?

The question has been raised as to whether fiber is useful for helping to control problems of overweight. Most dietary fiber, especially that in cereal grain, is hardly digested at all but rather passes through the system in a cleansing action that sweeps out the wastes efficiently. One has the filling satisfaction of eating amply, but little caloric weight can accumulate. However, there was little conclusive proof of the value of fiber for weight-control purposes until, in recent years, some of my colleagues and I set about designing some controlled experiments. So clear were the results that we can now safely claim that fiber, and specifically high-fiber bread, can play an important role in weight control.

There seems no question but that natural fiber must be included in any healthy diet. While regular cereals and fruits and vegetables provide some fiber, most of us can benefit by adding plain bran or high-fiber bread to ensure regularity and to diminish the chances of some serious diseases. It is an added advantage that fiber can help us control our weight, but it remains for me to show in the next chapter how this was proved. This concept is too new to stand without careful substantiation.

12

FIBER HELPS YOU LOSE WEIGHT, TOO

We have seen that dietary fiber is useful for regulating our body processes, that it is even vital for prevention of some of the most hazardous maladies of the Western world. There is another extraordinary advantage, though, that becomes important in our overweight society: Dietary fiber is a key to weight control.

An early pioneer in proving this was Dr. K. W. Heaton of the Bristol Royal Infirmary, Bristol, England. One of his experiments showed that volunteers eating whole-meal bread (which includes the bran) lost over three times as many calories in their daily body waste as volunteers eating the same amount of regular white bread. More calories passed right through the body system without adding to body weight (*Lancet*, December 22, 1973). That means that when we retain the natural fiber in bread we can enjoy eating more food and also have all the advantages of dietary fiber in prevention of disease. Or we can choose to lose weight without eating less food.

By 1973 Dr. Robert H. Cotton of ITT research labs in Rye, New York, was already pondering the question of improving regular white bread by adding dietary fiber. That would have the additional advantage of reducing the number of calories. At the lab, Stan Titcomb and Arty Juers had been developing a new, more wholesome bread that over the next three years was to overturn old concepts about the fattening effect of bread and shake up the diet world.

The new bread was 7.5 percent dietary fiber and had 30 percent fewer calories than regular bread. It had five times as much fiber as whole-wheat bread. In effect, two slices of the new bread would have as much fiber as ten slices of whole-wheat bread, or as much as two heaping bowls of all-bran cereal. And all the other nutrients in regular bread would still be there, plus increased calcium and iron.

Early on, as an independent consultant, I was asked to help design research that would test the safety and the weight-loss efficacy of the bread. At the time, this was a daring concept. Most dieters "know" they should cut down on bread and potatoes. One had to wonder if it would ever be possible to convince people that complex carbohydrate is an essential part of a balanced diet, and that you could lose weight effectively while eating substantial amounts of bread.

The Department of Food Science and Human Nutrition at Michigan State University contracted to carry out our experiments under the overall direction of Dr. Olaf Mickelson and with the direct supervision of Dr. D. D. Makdani. ITT supplied the high-fiber, reduced-calorie bread. I helped monitor the overall effort, helped organize the results and prepared some of the scientific papers that would document our conclusions and present them to the scientific community.

To ensure objectivity and credibility, it is often the case that university professors carry out research in cooperation with commercial companies. Ultimately, this research would have to pass muster with the Food and Drug Administration and the Federal Trade Commission, so any conclusions had to be proved by the highest standards possible. But you will judge that for yourself.

Sixteen overweight students were chosen at Michigan State University and put on an eight-week weight-control program, eating all their meals at a central cafeteria. All of them wanted to lose weight and all were supposed to be 10 to 25 pounds or more overweight.

THE EFFECTS OF DIETARY FIBER

They Could Eat as Much as They Liked

Volunteers could eat as much as they liked. There was no limit. But they were required to eat a minimum of 12 slices of bread a day and to avoid all alcoholic beverages. Calories in drinks are hard to measure unless specific shot glasses are used consistently. Any snacks consumed outside the cafeteria were to be recorded in a notebook so we could take that into account when we figured exactly what they all ate. On Sundays, volunteers were allowed a brown-bag lunch, premeasured and provided free, as were all their meals.

Of course, all volunteers were checked by a doctor, and they all signed consent forms. They were divided into two groups as evenly matched as possible. At random, one group was assigned to a regular bread diet and the other to a high-fiber bread diet, and no student ever knew which group he belonged to, or that the type of bread was the only difference between the two diets. The two breads look rather alike unless you compare them side by side and know what you are looking for. The high-fiber bread has a somewhat different texture.

To down as much as 12 slices a day, we had chosen only young men. Women rarely eat more than 5 or perhaps up to 8 slices a day. Their weight varies more too, increasing at the onset of menstruation. Also, in my experience, there is a curious fact about women: if they fall in love, they can lose weight with phenomenal ease and rapidity no matter what kind of food you put in front of them.

The other foods were foods typical of the American diet, not at all designed for weight loss. To prove our point about the efficacy of bread, and especially high-fiber bread, we gave them bacon, jelly, butter, whole milk and even cake, along with the eggs, meat and vegetables. This made it a bold experiment.

The young men were given 3200 calories a day on their cafeteria trays, regular cafeteria food but given high ratings for tastiness due to the special care. We certainly did not want them to go hungry. At each meal, along with butter, there was a cellophane package with 4 slices of bread. Each tray had the person's name, to be sure he got the right kind of bread and to allow the kitchen staff to weigh all leftovers. The lads quickly found that we were giving them too much food, and they did not like the idea of waste, so by common consent we reduced the menu to 2500 calories per day and told them they could always ask for more.

Even that was more than they cared to eat. Monitoring leftovers revealed that those eating regular bread averaged only 2343 calories per day. Admittedly, anybody who asked for second helpings would have raised the eyebrows of his colleagues. They had all agreed to try to lose weight, and Dr. Makdani himself attended most meals to lend support and observe the progress. A group spirit was developing under his warm encouragement and the volunteers did not want to let him down.

People on a High-Fiber Diet Ate Less Food

We mentioned the number of calories eaten by the users of regular bread. But one of the first startling facts to emerge was the difference in food consumption between that control group and the consumers of high-fiber bread. People on the high-fiber diet ate less food. Their average daily consumption was only 1972 calories, almost 400 calories less than the others.

Their 12 slices of high-fiber bread contained 216 fewer calories, but that still leaves 155 calories difference, which can be explained only by the fact that they felt less hungry without even knowing they were on a high-fiber diet. Random variation between the two groups cannot explain this difference. We must conclude that the fiber bread not only contains fewer calories but also satisfies the appetite better. The experimental group had cut down on their eating of other foods.

There was thus a double benefit to the high-fiber bread, aside from the usefulness of fiber in prevention of illness. Also, we were reassured to see that the reduction in eating was not in body-building protein, for there was a difference of only four grams a day in the average amount of protein they ate, and no difference in the absorption of protein. Those on the high-fiber diet consumed a little less fat and had a lower rate of absorption of fat in the digestive process.

Later, we were to confirm what others had found before us, that there was another significant advantage: The high-fiber group passed more calories through in their body waste, an additional benefit of 80 calories a day on the average. They thus had a total advantage of about 450 calories a day, which was reflected in the greater weight loss on the high-fiber diet.

Everyone Lost Weight on the Bread Diet

Everyone lost weight on the bread diet, even those eating regular bread. We did have three of the sixteen people drop out during the eight weeks, but even they lost weight as long as they remained with us.

One of the dropouts should not have been in the experiment at all; he was only 1.5 percent overweight. In the control group, he still lost 4¼ pounds in five weeks before giving up on us. I would not have wanted him to lose more.

Two in the test group dropped out; they were 28 to 34 percent overweight, weighing 200 pounds or more when they both should have weighed in the 160s. But both lost close to four pounds before abandoning us. The main reason for dropping was the inconvenience of taking all meals at a central cafeteria when living quarters and classrooms were widely dispersed. Certainly the diet regimen interfered with other activities.

I speak frankly about the dropouts. There are always some, and three is not many, as experiments go. But I do not want you to think we are reporting results from just a few successful dieters and forgetting about the relatively unsuccessful ones.

Over the eight weeks, the median weight loss was 16 pounds, or 2 pounds a week, a very sensible and successful amount. It meant that from 21 to 96 percent of the people's excess weight was trimmed away.

The young men had eaten adequately, even well, and yet had lost considerable weight. What explains this success? The bread, the lads said, satisfied any excess hunger. Also, the effect of a developing team spirit kept up morale and motivation under the kindly eye and encouragement of Dr. Makdani. The youths did not want to let him down. Too, they watched each other, and with weekly weighings and caliper measures of fat, they were kept informed by a constant check on progress.

In effect then, we proved that overweight young men could lose weight on a balanced and ample diet with heavy bread consumption if they are motivated and monitored carefully.

Fiber Helps Lose More Weight

All volunteers lost weight, but while those eating regular bread lost 13 pounds on the average, the test group, eating high-fiber bread, lost an average of 19 pounds in the eight-week-period. There was thus a 50 percent advantage to the high-fiber bread.

The control group on regular bread lost just over a quarter of their excess weight (median of 27 percent). The test group on high-fiber bread lost almost half of their excess weight (median loss of 46.5 percent of excess weight).

The results are very convincing, and with the help of my colleagues, I prepared a technical paper entitled, "Weight Loss with a Reduced-Calorie, High-Fiber Bread," which is being published under the authorship of O. Mickelson, D. D. Makdani, R. H. Cotton, S. T. Titcomb, J. C. Colmey, and myself. We document the weight-loss progress of each volunteer, show that there were no apparent problems of nitrogen or mineral balance, and give a full description of the experiment. Also, we show follow-up weighings to check on whether the program had lasting benefits.

Perhaps the severest test that any diet program faces is the matter of follow-up weighings to see if the weight loss is maintained. Ultimately, the problem is not so much how to lose weight as it is how to maintain the lower weight.

At the time this particular study ended, the high-fiber bread was not available in stores, but the young men were advised that they could continue the program with regular bread. However, when they were on their own, they would not have the disciplined mealtimes, monitored weekly weighings, or the group spirit that had kept morale high and supported their own will-power.

The formal experiment ended in June, 1974. It was clear that a few volunteers would promptly regain their lost weight. Some of them were perfectly open in talking about it. One young man spoke fondly of waiting for his first bout of martinis after two months on the wagon. A couple of others reveled in delight at the thought of Saturday beer parties to come. The omens were not all good for keeping those waistlines under control.

It was possible to weigh nine of the thirteen volunteers at the end of the summer, then six months later, and again after another six months. Four of the nine returned to the weight they had before the experiment; none of these men had continued to eat much bread at all. But five of the nine maintained most of their weight loss, or lost even more, and had not ignored the advantages of bread. Follow-up results are thus moderately encouraging.

Some people will persistently regard a diet as a temporary program, a "cure" rather than a sensible way of life. Bread, and especially reduced-calorie, high-fiber bread, does support a diet program effectively. Ultimately though, much depends on a person's firm commitment to continue the diet in the routine of everyday life, where bread may fit quite naturally.

All things considered, however, we still had not gone far enough with that one experiment. It is one thing to prove that a weight-loss program is possible under highly controlled conditions. It would be another thing to say that men and women of varying ages could follow a successful high-fiber bread diet in their own homes, without careful monitoring and daily encouragement. That was a matter for our next experiment.

The More Bread They Ate, the More Weight They Lost!

Our next experiment had a startling effect when results came to the attention of the media. "Let them eat bread! Watch them lose weight!'" was the title of a feature article in the usually conservative *Medical World News* (December, 1975). The *Chicago Tribune* announced, "Soon you'll be eating bread to lose weight." And spread across the front page in banner headlines, the not-so-conservative *National Enquirer* proclaimed, "The more bread you eat the more weight you lose" (March 9, 1976). This last striking headline was adapted from a sentence in one of my research reports: "I find convincing evidence that the more bread people ate, the more they lost weight."

Such apparently wild statements need a lot of substantiation. They rock the foundations of solidly entrenched misconceptions about the role of bread in a balanced diet and about any potential role of high-fiber bread in a weight-loss diet.

We already knew that this particular high-fiber bread was well received by people who like regular American bread. We knew it was a big help in a highly controlled weight-loss experiment. What we did not know was whether it could be used for controlling weight among families living and eating at home, without day-to-day monitoring. This time, also, we wanted a lot more people involved, of both sexes and of varying ages. Sixty-two volunteers were finally selected, again on a university campus, to participate in the next round. The volunteers were matched (keeping families together) according to the number of pounds they wished to lose, and were assigned to one of the groups that would each take a somewhat different approach to losing weight.

All were told they should decrease the amount of food eaten. They were briefed on the caloric content of various classes of foods and were advised to keep saturated fats to a minimum. The three groups were:

GROUP B: Bread Diet, twenty-one people. These people were given ample supplies of high-fiber bread and no guidance or instructions on how to follow a diet regimen.

GROUP B & BM: Bread Diet & Behavior Modification, twenty-two people. These people had ample supplies of the special bread, a behavior modification manual on how to design an individual weight-loss program, and access to weekly, supportive meetings under the guidance of Dr. Gordon Williams, psychologist. But there were no specific instructions on how to integrate the bread into a diet regimen.

GROUP BM: Behavior Modification, nineteen people. These people depended solely on the BM program with the manual and the weekly meetings.

Weights were recorded weekly, and at those times the groups receiving bread turned in diaries that recorded how much bread they had eaten each day. There was no other control over them, and no record of what other foods they ate, or how much they ate. They were on their own, except that the two BM groups had the weekly meetings if they cared to attend.

Only a Few People Did Not Succeed

Before we look at the remarkable success of the experiment, it is well to look for the moment to the people who did not succeed this time and who dropped from the experiment. Quite apparently, on some level, a few people think they should lose weight, but for one reason or another are not ready for the continuing commitment that weight control requires.

The Bread group was quite successful in this respect; of twenty-one people, only three dropped out during the eight weeks. This is a good record, probably only partly due to the fact that people were getting something for nothing. The bread diet seemed a natural thing that people could get used to.

The B & BM group was less successful in terms of dropouts; they lost seven out of twenty-two people. Apparently there was some confusion as to how to use the bread within the confines of the BM program. And admittedly, we gave them no help on this.

The BM group was scored also by as many as six out of nineteen people discontinuing the program. Possibly the disappointment over getting no free bread discouraged some. Others merely quit when they could not manage to lose weight as readily as they hoped. This different rate of dropouts moderates any direct comparison of weight loss among the three groups. But all groups were reasonably successful.

The B group alone accounted for an average loss of 4.3 pounds, the B & BM group 4.8 pounds and, for those who stayed with the BM group, there was an average loss of 8.31 pounds. But the average weight losses do not tell the whole story.

The Bread group had more consistent results throughout the group, a much lower amount of variation among the people. There was more variability from person to person with the B & BM group. And in the BM group, there was almost three times as much variance in weight loss among those who stayed through the whole eight weeks.

The story is that with the Behavior Modification program, for half of the people who stayed with it (six out of thirteen people), there was a very successful weight loss averaging 13.7 pounds. The others in that group had much more moderate success, and those who were not satisfied with their weight loss simply stopped coming in for the weekly weighings. The highly successful ones were also the highly motivated ones and, as neighbors, had given each other moral support and neighborly monitoring.

The most startling conclusion of this experiment was the fact that among the people using the high-fiber bread, the more bread they ate, the more weight they lost.

Routinely checking if weight loss was related to the amount of bread eaten, I was amazed at what the computer kept telling me. I could hardly believe it: Volunteers lost an average of half a pound of weight per week for every additional slice of bread they ate each day, over the two-month period. This shows up when you run a trend line through the data. The computer also told me that this half pound is statistically significant, though I still insist it is a very crude estimate. (My computer and I do not always see eye to eye on matters of judgment.) But let us see how the computer could come up with such a remarkable result.

The median bread consumption was an average of 7.3 slices a day. Those who ate less bread lost an average of four pounds.

More bread consumed gave an average loss of six pounds. When we rank the people by how much bread they consumed, we find that the top 25 percent lost 6.1 pounds, the next 25 percent lost 5.7 pounds, and so on. The quartile of people who ate the least bread lost 4.4 pounds.

This is, of course, only a brief account of the whole experiment. I wrote up the detailed study in a technical paper called, "Home Dieting with Reduced-Calorie, High-Fiber Bread and Behavior Modification." This is being published under the authorship of O. Mickelson, myself, D. D. Makdani, G. Williams, R. H. Cotton and J. C. Colmey.

Food chemists were first to learn the details of our experiment at the 61st Annual Meeting of the American Association of Cereal Chemists in New Orleans, in October 1976. There our colleague Stan Titcomb described our work and the success of the product that he had developed.

It was early in the next year, in March 1977, that the National Institutes of Health invited our people to present our findings at a medical and nutritional conference on "The Role of Dietary Fiber in Health," at Bethesda, Maryland. A special workshop was featured there on fiber and the overweight problem, and our work was presented to the medical community by Dr. John Colmey and Stan Titcomb.

By this time, the unusual discovery had been reviewed by several leading experts. Theodore Van Itallie, M.D., of Columbia University's Medical School and St. Luke's Hospital Center, devoted a meeting of his Metabolism Seminar to hearing a presentation by Dr. Colmey. At the Mayo Clinic in Rochester, Minnesota, P. J. Palumbo, M.D., and his associates conducted their own research, and he wrote, "I am impressed with the weight reduction that is accomplished with high-fiber bread." From his own experiments, and after further review of our work, he wrote that "it may indeed be appropriate . . . to recommend a diet high in unavailable carbohydrate for the general population in order to control serum lipid levels and to control obesity."

Other research was carried out by Hans Kaunitz, M.D., clinical professor emeritus at Columbia University's College of Physicians and Surgeons. He reported, "We have been using reduced-calorie bread for over two years in the treatment of overweight patients. Our experience has been very encouraging, particularly when we tried to maintain reduced weight."

Working with ten patients who had achieved their desired weight, Dr. Kaunitz reports, "They have been able to maintain reduced weight over protracted periods." He was particularly impressed that the fiber in the special bread gives a feeling of having eaten enough and also counteracts the usual tendency to constipation that people often suffer when on a reduced-calorie diet.

After we had proved the safety and efficacy of the product as an aid to weight loss, the crucial question was whether the fiber bread can help keep the weight off as part of an everyday, continuing diet that people can live with and enjoy. Many overweight people can lose weight, but they cannot always keep things that way. Our own work, and especially the work of Dr. Kaunitz, seems to indicate that high-fiber bread is a useful part of an ongoing program of weight control.

The bread itself, of course, does not directly cause weight loss. Without motivation, without some other caloric restrictions, the special bread, or any other fiber product, will not make you lose weight.

Given the motivation to control weight in a lasting change of life-style, you will find the fiber bread can be a big help. And, as we have shown, even regular bread can play a useful role.

Part Five

LIVING WITH A WEIGHT-CONTROL PLAN

13

HOW TO CHANGE YOUR EATING HABITS PERMANENTLY

Clearly, if research has taught us anything about weight control, it has taught us that a diet for weight control must be a diet for living. It has to include a lasting, livable change of life-style if the weight loss is to be maintained.

This means that our attitudes and behavior must change and stay changed. But how does one do that? The techniques were hardly conceived of before fifteen years ago, and have been refined only in very recent years. Just making a decision to follow a diet program is not usually enough to last for long unless people can see progressive results and can map out a strategy for maintaining the impetus until it becomes second nature. That strategy is what we are talking about here.

When and Where Temptation Lurks

First off, it is a good idea to anticipate the various places and times of temptation so that you will have an advance plan for being on your guard. Each person's environment is a little different, but we can list the major places and times that could affect you.

1. When you are shopping: The danger is that you will buy more food than your family needs, and be tempted to buy some of the wrong kinds of food, especially if they are on sale or are displayed attractively in the store. The best idea is to plan your week's meals ahead and to use a shopping list carefully made up in advance. If you want to take advantage of sale items, do so by advance planning. Advertisements in the local newspapers often announce by Wednesday what will be on sale on Friday and Saturday. In some places, like New York State, the Department of Agriculture keeps track of prices and quality, sending out news releases or newsletters on good buys. New York City even has a phone number to give current nutrition tips, in accord with the season and the market supply of produce, meats, poultry, and dairy foods. If you happen to see tempting sales or discounts when in the grocery store, pass them by if they are not on your list. Saving money that way is being penny wise and pound foolish, in terms of the temptation to eat what you have bought at a bargain. It is no bargain if you collect the pounds at your midriff. Food kept out of your house is that much less food to tempt you.

One trick is to take shopping only enough money for what you need, as best as you can guess it. Also, shop after you have eaten, so that any appetite of the moment is less likely to influence you into overbuying. Leaving the children at home, if possible, is another way of keeping unneeded food from finding its way into your shopping basket and then into your home. Husbands, too, if they are not the regular shoppers in the family, tend to overspend and buy on impulse. Also, they are generally less concerned about weight control and the fattening effects of certain foods.

2. If someone offers you food: A neighbor may bring a cake or home-baked brownies. You should find a way of declining. A firm "Thanks, but no thanks," with a friendly smile, and perhaps a word or two (no more, it's a bore to others) about your new weight-control life-style. Act just the way an ex-smoker would if offered a cigarette: a very firm no, a rejection of the thing, and not of the person.

Last week a new graduate student came to my home for an early morning appointment and happened to bring some Danish pastry for us both. "I thought you might like to have some breakfast," he said. "They are fresh, I just got them on the way here this morning." I thanked him for his kindness. He meant well. Then it seemed to come to him. "It's not the kind of thing I suppose I should bring to someone writing a diet book," he said awkwardly. My smile was supportive of him, but not of his pastry. When he left, I suggested, "Perhaps you would like to take the pastry along," but it is not easy to take back a little gift. He demurred and left them. Of course I could then have given them to someone else, perhaps a poor person in Greenwich Village, where I live. But the important thing for me was to get them out of my home fast. They went into the incinerator within minutes after he left.

What a waste, you may think. But I am surely not a human garbage pail, and my eating them would not help either me or the famished people of India. Particularly those of us who grew up in the Depression or the Second World War have to *learn* to throw out excess food from our homes. My view is that its very presence is a danger. It is as simple as saying that if it is not there you can't make the mistake of eating it. We ought to be more concerned about our waists than we are about our waste.

3. In the kitchen: You will do well to throw out surplus perishable food and any junk food (most things high in sugar, salt, saturated fat, or calories).

A dietary scale for weighing portions should be handy on the kitchen table or counter at all times. So much the better if it shows grams as well as ounces, because the United States is moving inexorably and fairly fast to the metric system of measurement. But the idea is not only to have the scale handy, but to use it for weighing virtually everything you are going to eat. Do not trust yourself to guess until you have had a few months of experience and are really settled into your new life-style. Then it's still a good idea to weigh everything, just to be sure. You develop the habit of weighing, counting, and measuring so that unconscious errors cannot creep in, and you are automatically on guard against slips.

You will also need a handy set of measures: cup, half-cup,

third-cup, quarter-cup, tablespoon, and teaspoon, and you should keep in mind always that these are level measures, not for heaping and overflowing.

Other people in your family may do some cooking, or keep some of their own favorite foods and snacks around. You know this, but now you should carefully identify the dangers. There may be crackers, cookies, cupcakes, candy bars, cold cuts, mayonnaise. Whatever these things are, try to keep them out of the way, separate and identified, as inaccessible as possible. It is fair to enlist the help of others in the family to keep junk foods out of the house, or in the case of children, to enforce a ban when persuasion fails. At the very least, a certain shelf of the kitchen cupboard or part of the refrigerator can be reserved for other peoples' weaknesses, and in your mind you mark off that area as forbidden territory for you. If some of your family insists on fattening foods or junk foods, let them prepare it themselves; you don't have to be an accomplice to their nutritional crimes. You can't usually stop a person from eating unwisely in your home, but you shouldn't have to help them in their self-destructiveness. Just have them keep it out of your way.

While cooking we all occasionally taste the things we are making. That is a danger point. I know more than one overweight housewife who eats very lightly at meals, in front of her family—and likes to have them notice that she eats very little —but she has sampled so much of her own cooking in the kitchen, she hardly needs a meal to follow that. The answer? Don't taste unless you really have to. Use the nose instead of the mouth to sense the right flavor. But if taste you must, use the smallest teaspoon or fork you have. Or better yet, get someone else to do the tasting. Whether or not something is cooked enough may be tested better by inserting a knife or by just looking at it, rather than by eating a piece of it.

Fussing about in the kitchen, it is all too easy to pop things into the mouth. It is a good idea to put food away promptly and keep any nibbling to preplanned snacks when you know exactly what you are doing. In other words, never ever nibble in the kitchen. Very strictly it is a place for preparing food, not for eating it.

4. At the table: Your meal table may be in the kitchen, and it may even be the same table where you prepare the food. Nonetheless, make a distinction. When you are preparing food, you do not eat. When you eat, even if it's a preplanned snack, you clear off any food that is not a planned part of the meal, you sit down when you eat, you do nothing else: no newspapers or book, no TV, no diversion at all unless it is family conversation. Even with family conversation, it is best to be conscious of each mouthful of food, and to put the fork down between bites, to chew slowly, to eat slowly and very deliberately, enjoying the taste.

Overweight people tend to be fast eaters, so slow yourself down deliberately, perhaps beginning your meal a few minutes after others have started. Consider starting with a glass of plain water, sipping slowly and taking your time. Part of the danger of fast eating is that your body system needs about twenty minutes from the time it has had enough to signal that feeling to your conscious mind. If you eat too fast, you may finish the meal still feeling hungry, only because you haven't yet got the signal of satiety. So eat slowly, chew carefully, and enjoy your food! If there is fruit or dessert at the end of a meal, wait at least ten minutes before you begin it. That gives more time for your system to recognize that you have had enough.

No seconds should appear on the table, no serving bowls from which you might be tempted to take a little more. If there are leftovers from the cooking, try to pack them in individual portions so that you can take out one portion at a time. All food should be served on separate plates for each person, and what another person leaves uneaten should not tempt you to help him. No one should be a human disposal system for leftovers! Throw it out with aplomb, even with pride, or quickly store it in the refrigerator, as far away as possible from temptation, preferably frozen so that it can't be consumed conveniently or casually.

Sometimes you will have guests at your table, and that raises some special challenges. You want to put out a good spread, but you are probably also tempted to fill the plates amply and to bring second helpings. Well, quality cooking is fine, and ample servings are all right for your guests, if that is what they really want. But not for you, if it is an evening meal. Most of the time no one will notice what you have on your plate, or how much— and if they do, what does it matter? Nothing and no one should bend your will. You can be proud of yourself for keeping careful control, all the more careful when guests and extra foods are around. For both you and your guests, you can practice the art of filling the plate with little food. Lettuce leaves, pickles, parsley, tomato—all help make the plate look full while it carries a modest caloric load.

5. **When you are a guest at someone's home:** At such times the challenge can be even more intense. The hostess looks hurt if you don't take second helpings, or you decline to taste the calorie-rich dessert she has prepared. It is all too easy to be intimidated into eating more than you need or want. It may take practice, but you will have to learn to say a pleasant but firm "No, thank you," that shows not a flicker of wavering. (Some people say no in a weak way that invites more urging from the host or hostess; they protest all the way to their acceptance.) Your answer has to be clear-cut and definite. Beforehand, it might be helpful to advise your hostess that you eat very lightly in the evening and that you are on a weight-control program. Enlist her sympathetic support and she may be more considerate, but never be shaken in your resolve, no matter how much pressure people put on you. Having a supportive spouse can be a big help.

There is less trouble than you might think in saying no. Years ago I gave up alcohol, and most other useless or dangerous foods and beverages. When cocktails are served it is easy to ask for plain club soda, or a diet soft drink. At the table I turn my wineglass upside down and hardly have to say a word of refusal: the message is clear. Someone is passing the hors d'oeuvre tray, and you either let it pass or pick out an innocent radish and let it go. If someone pours you a drink, just put it down somewhere and leave it. And don't be afraid to leave food on the plate. What your hostess wants is a compliment more than a clean plate, so it can ease the situation to be sure and notice out loud what is really tasty and attractive, without implying you want more.

6. **In a restaurant:** Meals at a restaurant can be as much of a challenge or more than eating at someone's home. You can't control the portion size served, but you can control what you choose. Automatically it is easiest if you skip the cocktail, the hors d'oeuvres, and dessert, and settle for a main course. Keep your hand out of the bread basket, except for what your meal plan allows, and treat the butter dish the way you would a plate of arsenic, unless your weight is well under control, and you are entitled to the maintenance supplement.

Some restaurants give you a free glass of wine or liqueur, or all the beer you can drink, included in the price. It is hard to turn down something for free, but that's what you have got to do in most cases. Your host may urge upon you the biggest steak, the most caloric dessert, and you have got to plan ahead on being extra careful to pass it up instead of putting it on in terms of weight. The price of liberty from fat is constant vigilance, recognizing in advance these dangerous situations and being prepared for them, most especially in the evening.

If you may lunch at work, there should be no problem if you or your spouse prepares a brown bag carefully. Cafeteria food usually includes tuna salads and light dishes, with plenty of fruit. More dangerous is the local delicatessen or sandwich shop, with overloads of mayonnaise, potato salad, and high-cholesterol, fatty cold cuts. Best bets there might be a salmon sandwich (small, whole can of salmon) or tuna, holding the mayo, and avoiding shrimp, tuna, or salmon salad, which is high in calories and low in protein. Breast of turkey or chicken is a good bet, followed by fruit. It is horrifying how many people pick up a candy bar with lunch, or instead of lunch. I see that often with youngsters, especially girls who are watching their weight. Hopefully they will learn better before too much damage is done. It's rather a shame that vending machines used for snacks or lunch seem to sell either junk foods, dull, stale sandwiches, or coffee without flavor.

7. **The coffee break:** This is another dangerous time. So-called Danish pastry is a menace to good nutrition and to the waistline, too. Junk food carried by most coffee shops and coffee wagons that roll around offices adds rolls around your middle. Tea or black coffee is fine, and it is an excellent idea to take a piece of fruit as an energy pickup. Any food snack must be part and parcel of the dietary meal plan, and while it is advisable to plan for both midmorning and midafternoon snacks, impulse snacking is a lethal seduction to which the answer must be a very firm no. It is no virtue to skip a planned meal or snack. Quite the contrary. If you go without food in the morning, or at lunch, you will pay for it later by urges to eat and eat in the evening, when the calories do most harm. Breakfast, particularly, is the most important meal of the day. Nutritionist Ethel Maslansky, now retired, spent years with New York City's public health clinics, helping people to control their weight. She herself has known what it is to have to lose weight, and when I asked her to sum up what, in her experience, was most important in weight-loss success, she explained it in terms of herself with advice she thinks can apply to anyone. "I do have to have a good breakfast. Then I am comfortable all day. Then the most important thing is having a snack between meals. I'm never so hungry that I lose control. I can moderate the meals as long as I have snacks during the day—not in the evening."

8. **The critical time of danger is in the evening, and especially late at night:** The late night urge to eat is so dangerous that Albert J. Stunkard, Professor of Neurological Sciences at the University of Pennsylvania, has referred to it as the "night-eating syndrome." At that time the body rhythms are in a different state than in the morning. Even a small snack can trigger an uncontrollable eating binge that is hard to stop.

It is well known that overweight people are capable of not eating (many unwisely skip breakfast); their difficulties lie in how to stop eating once they have started, especially at night. At that time, their defenses are down and they don't so readily perceive body signals telling them to quit. The answer has got to be a self-imposed strict rule never to touch even the smallest amount of food after a light and early supper. If the oral urge is strong and you are impatient for the urge to pass (as it will, according to your ninety-minute body rhythm), then a glass of water or plain soda will satisfy it as well as a box of cookies, and you will feel much less guilty. Recognizing this time as deadly dangerous should help keep you on guard, aware of the weakness, and defended against it.

Curiously enough, people find that physical activity alleviates any urgent appetite. A walk is as good as a meal to satisfy the urge. And, for reasons that are unknown to science, a hot bath will pamper your body system into forgetting that it was tempting you to eat.

Monitor Yourself with a Daily Diary

The eating urge should never catch you unaware. To identify the danger times and keep a check on progress, the best single idea that has emerged from psychological research is the keeping of a daily diary.

Don't think for a minute that this is childish. Behavioral research has shown that it helps a great deal in weight control and also in programs to reduce and then eliminate the smoking habit. At Baruch College, City University of New York, we have a Body Clock Diet Club that includes faculty as well as students, and even a few alumni. They have lost just under a ton of weight by following these ideas, and they have helped me develop the techniques.

The diary should be first of all a plan, made a week in advance, showing what will be eaten when. On one page is the day's diet plan, with space to check off each item that is eaten, according to plan. Any substitutions—occasionally necessary because of eating out, or because of unavailability of the planned food—are written in, along with the time of day to the nearest hour. Always, dinner is limited to no more than 30 percent of the day's calories, and breakfast should contain at least as many calories as lunch. Remember that if you have trouble swallowing solid food in the morning, you can take your calories in nutritious liquid form as a high-protein drink, along with dietary fiber in the form of unprocessed bran or high-fiber bread, and fruit, which may also be blended into the beverage.

Besides food plans and actual eating behavior, the daily page should show the exercise plan and the check-off, or substitution, of the actual exercise taken. The exercise—daily, if at all possible—is about as important as the regulation of eating. Repeatedly, research has shown that overweight people are distinguished more by inactivity than by overeating. And the exercise should be aerobic, giving rise to a gentle sweat and working the heart and lungs at a moderate pace that will bring the body into condition without any dangerous strain.

Some of our people at Baruch College have rated how they feel before exercise, and then how they feel after it. Inevitably, the rating rises dramatically. They use the seven-point mood scale we have described, going from (1) depressed, "blue" to (7) happy, elated.

Numbers cannot, however, reflect the range and varieties of your feelings, which are vitally important to controlled and carefully timed eating. You will need space on the daily diary for recording your feelings with a word or two: "lonely," "feel unappreciated," "self-confident," "frustrated," "angry," "active," "tired," "bored." These are quite as important as "hungry" or "eating urge." You will see how often you think you are hungry, or have an urge to eat, when your feelings are down. That is not food hunger, it is emotional hunger! Seeing this, repeated through the days, will let you see that much of your eating has been for emotional reasons and not for nutrition or even for enjoyment.

Reward Yourself for Success

It is hardly worthwhile to monitor your weight on a daily basis. That suggests too much impatience for short-term results. Day by day you follow the program, and it is significant to check on your progress each week at the same time, wearing as few clothes as possible. Some weeks you will be delighted with a greater loss than you expected, some weeks your weight may appear to be hardly changed. The body seems to have set-points, as if it preferred certain levels of weight, and there is no reason to be discouraged at this. They are natural plateaux and they will be overcome if you just continue steadily and with confidence. Perhaps the greatest potential enemy of your success is an impatience for instant results, discouragement at the first sign that you read as the diet's not effecting immediate wonders with the waistline and weight. The very human temptation is to expect a magic that will whisk the pounds off and then let you forget about continued weight control as a way of life. That is an unrealistic and medically dangerous fantasy. What you need is a quiet confidence that you are doing the right thing and the realization that you cannot fail as long as you treat yourself and food with a new respect and maintain a constant vigilance for moments of weakness.

Meanwhile, it helps to savor the rewards of success. The weight you are aiming for can be marked prominently in the diary and seen not just as a number of pounds, but as the symbol of your goal, felt with all the pleasure that the new look and feeling of self-control will bring.

A helpful aid to that goal is a good supplemental reward for stages in your progress. Our Baruch College Diet Club has found it useful to plan a really impressive reward for yourself at the halfway mark toward reaching your desired weight. Then another, larger reward after you have maintained your goal weight for one week. That is, the reward is not only for success, but finally for maintained success, when you have had a week of showing that you intend to keep the excess weight off your body.

Any weight-loss program that is to be medically safe and successful must concentrate on keeping the weight off, not just on losing it.

The reward you must pick yourself, and you must award it yourself, because the purpose is to please yourself. You are losing weight for you and for how you feel about yourself, not for others and how they feel about you. Just maintaining a good self-image can be aided by family, friends, spouse, or lover, but it should never be dependent on or bound to others' views of you, or their appreciation of the New You. Choose a vacation you have always wanted, a new dress that will do justice to your figure, even a new car or a television, if you can afford it. It doesn't have to be something that costs money. It can be as simple as setting aside time for yourself, away from other obligations, doing something just because it pleases you.

Help from Others

Help from others, of course, is a great aid, and there is nothing the matter with enlisting the support of friends or family in holding to your program of weight control. Your immediate family may or may not be helpful. (Some people close to us can, for whatever reasons, sometimes undermine our confidence, instead of helping us.) Then it is a good idea to turn to other friends outside the home. In moments of weakness, with the pressing urge to eat, danger can be averted by a phone call to some supportive friend, with no motive needed other than a call for a few words of moral support. Often just talking about the problem will alleviate it. Don't feel silly or self-conscious about calling for help and saying that is what you are calling for. There is a power to be tapped in other people's strength when we are at a low ebb in the rhythms of our self-confidence and strength of purpose.

This basic technique of phoning for moral support is used by many self-help groups, including many diet clubs, as well as SmokeEnders, Alcoholics Anonymous, and Gamblers Anonymous. They are all concerned with handling destructive habits and compulsive urges, and they all lean heavily on someone to turn to who really understands the problem and the temptation. Somehow, a strength emerges from sharing the problem and the success that cannot be achieved by an individual alone.

Again, don't be embarrassed, aloof, or too shy to use this technique. It works, and curiously enough, it helps you if others call you for help. You will find strength in giving strength to others. Basically, it breaks the dangerous isolation of the individual, who may become discouraged and feel very much alone with the problem, as if he or she were unique in having periodic swings of weakness in the face of compulsive urges. Only a false pride can keep you from reaching for the phone and a friend.

Family or personal friends may not be sympathetic or, more likely, may just be unable to understand the plight of the overeater. "Why don't you just stop when you have had enough?" is the kind of comment that can drive fat people out of their skulls and practically cause remission.

There is no question in my mind of the benefit of diet clubs such as Overeaters Anonymous (OA), Take Off Pounds Sensibly (TOPS), or the commercial equivalents such as Weight Watchers. Locally, you should check what is available. Some companies or colleges have their own groups. Even the commercial groups do not cost much in light of their worth in giving you support. Only be careful because these organizations are not necessarily informed on the latest advances in diet research, like the advantages of fiber in the diet, or, most especially, the importance of an ample breakfast and a meager evening meal.

My strong advice is to join one of these groups and take the time to attend them frequently. What is more important in your life than your basic health and controlling your weight? Just hearing about the problem and talking about it can bring a renewed sense of purpose, and identification with others brings with it a strong resolve in changing your life-style.

You may have to find the right group for you. They differ in approach, and in social background of the members. But do not go to criticize; go to learn and to benefit by sharing the experience of weight loss. Other people's successes will encourage you to realize that it can be done, when you are inclined to doubt your progress. Most overweight people have been overweight for years, and even during previous crash dieting, have developed entrenched eating attitudes and behaviors that favor fatness.

It is easy, in a sense, to know what one ought to do to control weight: Balanced nutrition is a necessity for good health, as are control of the amount of food, and emphasis on when you eat as well as what foods you eat. Exercise is essential, and aerobic exercise particularly helpful. You know, as I say, what ought to be done. The real challenge is to implement the advice and retain ongoing motivation while new habits are replacing the old. This takes obedience to simple rules discovered by behavioral scientists, and it is greatly helped by sharing the experience with others. Your own success is likely to give hope to others and instill in you the significance of your own accomplishment so that you will never lose hold of that new way of life.

14

THE NEW YOU AND HOW TO STAY
THAT WAY

You can have the utmost confidence that you will lose weight with the Body Clock Diet, especially when you control the type and the amount of food you eat, and if you take aerobic exercise regularly. It is really easy when you get on the right track.

Even if you can't bring yourself to eat less, and you can't get started with an exercise plan, there will be a significant weight-reducing advantage to shifting the bulk of your eating away from the evening and making sure you eat an ample breakfast to start the day. By controlling when you eat, you can fine-tune your system to take off (or put on) the amount of weight you like. That is the ultimate power of the Body Clock Diet.

Your body is not to be treated as an impersonal machine. You must learn to feel and sense the natural rhythms of the body. Go with the rhythms, and come to know that it feels right when you have learned to eat (or drink) an ample breakfast, and gone light at night.

"At first the idea horrified me, of sitting down to a heavy meal in the morning. I didn't feel like it, and didn't have the time anyway," says Betty H., an anthropology student from Seattle. "The only way I would take any breakfast was to try that idea of the high-protein drink, whipped up in a blender. That was easy enough and quick enough. Then, gradually, somehow, I found I was feeling better. More energy, better moods. And now in the evening, I don't get so hungry. It seems natural to eat light when my body doesn't need the food." Betty has found that 22 pounds have slipped away, mainly by cutting down on the heavy dinners she used to eat in the evening. "I like my food," she went on, "but I just had to learn to like it in the morning. I used to skip breakfast and think I was being virtuous, but later at night, I seemed to get out of control. Now it's all so easy, as long as I get a good breakfast and stay away from junk foods."

You Don't Feel Like Eating So Much in the Evening

There is a natural reduction in how much you eat because you don't feel like eating so much in the evening when you have had a good breakfast. It is well, though, to watch very carefully the amounts you eat, very especially in the evening. Destructive overeating in the evening has been part of your life for a long time, and you may need several weeks to find the changeover easy.

Mid-morning and mid-afternoon snacks help keep energy levels high during the day. It is an easy matter to save one of the fruits from your breakfast or lunch to have at this time, or use high-fiber bread or toast. If you have been at your goal weight for a week or more, you may choose this in-between time for your supplemental allowance (up to 150 calories), but no caloric snacks are to be taken at night, only the relatively non-caloric foods and beverages I have listed.

One hundred years ago, gourmet Brillat-Savarin said that we are what we eat. Now we can say "We are not only what we eat, but *when* we eat." This new insight was reported at the 2nd International Congress on Energy Balance in Man. And indeed, it is a special kind of energy crisis that we face. With food as fuel for body energy, we must learn how to refuel our bodies by eating when excess food is least likely to be stored in the form of fat.

We individually are not responsible for our own tendency to

conserve energy in the form of fat. Some people were born with an all-too-thrifty body that stores up fat readily and is reluctant to exercise. But if you are that type, remember it is not your fault, for you did not choose the genes you were born with. There should be no blame or shame in being fat, for it is not a moral issue. Society will be slow to recognize this, but it is vital that you recognize it and not feel guilty about your own condition. You can still work to get rid of the excess fat, but do it on your own terms, for yourself, and for how you feel about yourself—never out of shame or guilt.

There's no sense either in feeling guilty or wasteful over leaving food on your plate, refusing food, or even throwing it out. Anything to avoid the temptation to eat it. Remember what I said about not being a human garbage pail, or a helpless victim of other people's misguided hospitality. Your pride in yourself will see you through; guilt never will.

Remember the Rewards

It helps always to keep in mind the rewards that accrue to the New You when you maintain control of your eating behavior and your weight. Savor these benefits so you know it is worthwhile, and appreciate them every day.

1. You look better and feel more attractive and youthful. You notice it and others notice it, too. Don't take it for granted. Enjoy it and know that it is the result of your own controlled eating behavior.

2. You feel better; your body tone is better and your basic health is better. Chances are you will live longer, too, and be free of many of the ailments of modern society, especially if you add fiber to your meals each day. Following the Body Clock Diet, you are more likely to be spared the knockout of illnesses— saved by the clock, in a manner of speaking.

3. A better appearance is a definite asset socially, but it is also an economic asset. When your weight is under control,

people respect you more and are more likely to see you as having ability on the job. Studies have shown that thin people are paid more than fat people; they are respected more; they are treated better.

4. You will find that you can do more. It is not just a matter of self-confidence, but also a question of energy and inclination to be active. The slender person can do more with less effort and so is likely to accomplish more.

5. Given the opportunity, your sex life is likely to improve greatly. Certainly your ability and interest will. Hilde Bruch, one authority on weight-loss control, reports that most of her overweight patients have remarkably little sexual interest. Dr. Richard E. Nisbett, Associate Professor at the University of Michigan, discovered that obese college students had fewer orgasms than other students. And Dr. Alex Comfort of London's University College comments, "What isn't realized is that in men overweight is a physical cause of impotence." Apparently it is a matter of using it or losing it: all the more reason to maintain your new life-style if you value your sex life as well as your life, to turn a phrase from *The Joy of Sex*. An added benefit, of course, is the 150 calories or so that you burn off when you make love.

All this and more is yours for the having in a new life-style of slenderness. The self-confidence that emerges will infuse your whole personality and run through every part of your life. In the words of one woman, "We begin to use our newfound strength to cope with other problems, too."

Remember always that you are never too hurried to have breakfast, and one that includes plenty of protein. Natalie A., a young bank executive who puts in a ten-hour day and commutes to work, says, "The very fact that I am so busy and hurried makes it all the more important to start the day with energy ready in reserve. When things are really hectic, I depend on a sugar-free, high-protein drink, blended with fruit in a base of skim milk, with a little fiber added." That way, Natalie can have over one-third of her day's calories before leaving for work. She feels better, and easily keeps her figure trim. "I don't ever want to see again those fifteen pounds that I lost. It's such a great thing to look forward to summer when I'll be proud of my figure in a bathing suit. I bought a new bikini and might even dare to wear it."

Impulsive urges to eat when you shouldn't may still strike from time to time, but you will be well prepared to meet them head on. You know now, from your food diary, when those urges come, the time of day. or night, and the kind of situation that prompts them. You know the urge will pass if you turn your mind to something else, and even more especially if you stay physically active. If the urge rages at you or nags, a glass of water, a cup of tea or bouillon will usually pacify it. Food is no longer your emotional support or crutch, and you are not afraid of occasionally feeling the edge of an appetite that adds a little zest to life, instead of pounds of fat.

Eat as Many Chocolate Sundaes as You Like

Feeling an eating urge, especially at night, is as much an opportunity as a problem. If you can't chase it away, indulge it more than fully with your fantasy. Think of this: You can eat as many chocolate sundaes as you want—tomorrow morning. You can wade into a box of crackers and cheese, go on to enjoy a steak and demolish all the wild desserts you can dream of. But not right now. Tomorrow morning. Enjoy, if you like, all the pleasant anticipation and the abandon of reverie. But don't act on it for now.

Tomorrow morning you will very probably find the mad desires of the night-eating craze have passed. You can settle easily for an ample and healthily nutritious breakfast, which is what you need in the morning. Everything is in the art of postponing a little, not in total denial for all time. That is too forbidding, too long, and too negative a promise to keep. Promise yourself anything, but postpone it till breakfast, when, it so happens, the light of day will put things in a bright new perspective.

193

LIVING WITH A WEIGHT-CONTROL PLAN

We live most fully a day at a time, feeling the pulse of life through the daily rhythms of the body and mind. Those days will add up to equal a lifetime of health and weight control. The best kind of dieting is like the best kind of love: It is lived each day, but it lasts a lifetime.

REFERENCES

Chapter 3. It Is Not Your Fault You Are Fat!

Bray, G. A., and J. E. Bethune, eds., *Treatment and Management of Obesity*. New York: Harper and Row, 1974, 149 pp.

Mann, G. V., "The Influence of Obesity on Health." *New England Journal of Medicine*, July 25, 1974, pp. 178–185, and August 1, 1974, pp. 226–232.

Mayer, J., *Overweight: Causes, Cost, and Control*. Englewood Cliffs, N.J.: Prentice-Hall, Inc., 1968, 213 pp.

Miller, D. S., and S. Parsonage, "Resistance to Slimming: Adaptation or Illusion?" *Lancet*, April 5, 1975, pp. 773–775.

Chapter 4. Getting Started: How Much Do You Want to Weigh?

Durnin, J. V. G. A., and M. M. Rahaman, "The Assessment of the Amount of Fat in the Human Body from Measurements of Skinfold Thickness." *British Journal of Nutrition* 21 (1967):681.

McGanity, W. J., and W. J. Darby. "Some Considerations in Making Therapeutic Trials," in H. Spector, *et al.*, eds., *Methods for Evaluation of Nutritional Adequacy and Status*. Office of the Quartermaster General, U.S. Department of the Army NA 22:N95/2 (December 1954):82–88.

"New Weight Standards for Men and Women." Metropolitan Life Insurance Company Statistical Bulletin, vol. 40, no. 1 (November–December 1959).

REFERENCES

Chapter 5. If You Can't Wait for Gradual Results

Blackburn, G. L., B. R. Bistrian, and J.-P. Flatt, "Role of a Protein-Sparing Fast in a Comprehensive Weight Reduction Programme." *Recent Advances in Obesity Research.* London: Newman, 1975.

Bloom, W. L., "Fasting as an Introduction to the Treatment of Obesity." *Metabolism* 8 (1959):214–220.

Drenick, E. J., "Weight Reduction by Prolonged Fasting." *Medical Times* 100 (January 1972):209–229.

Keckwick, A., and G. L. S. Powan, "Metabolic Studies in Human Obesity with Isocaloric Diet High in Fat, Protein, and Carbohydrate." *Metabolism* 6 (1957):447.

"'Protein-Sparing': New Option for Nutritional Support." *Hospital Practice* (December 1976):88–90.

Yang, M.-u., and T. B. Van Itallie, "Composition of Weight Lost During Short-Term Weight Reduction." *Journal of Clinical Investigation* 58 (September 1976):722–730.

Chapter 6. Exercise Is an Essential Part of the Commitment

Gwinup, G., "Effects of Diet and Exercise in the Treatment of Obesity," in G. A. Bray and J. E. Bethune, eds., *Treatment and Management of Obesity.* New York: Harper & Row, 1974, pp. 93–102.

Payne, P. R., E. F. Wheeler, and C. B. Salvosa, "Prediction of Daily Energy Expenditure from Average Pulse Rates." *American Journal of Clinical Nutrition* 24 (September 1971):1164–1170.

Thomas, D. W., and J. Mayer, "The Search for the Secret of Fat." *Psychology Today,* September 1973, pp. 74–79.

Chapter 7. These People Lost Weight by Eating Their Meals Earlier!

Graeber, R. C., R. Gatty, F. Halberg, and H. Levine, *Human Eating Behavior: Preferences, Consumption Patterns, and Biorhythms.* Natick, Massachusetts: U. S. Army Research and Development Command, Food Science Laboratories Technical Report (final report in contract DAAK03–74–c–0233), in press, 1978.

Graeber, R. C., and F. Halberg, "You Are When You Eat." Paper presented at the annual meeting of the Eastern Psychological Association, New York City, April 1976, 18 pp.

Halberg, F., "Implications of Biological Rhythms for Clinical Practice." *Hospital Practice,* January 1977, pp. 139–149.

REFERENCES

Halberg, F., and B. Sullivan, "Meal Schedules and Their Inter-action with the Body's Schedules." Proceedings of the 10th International Congress on Nutrition, Kyoto, Japan, August 1975; abstracted in *Chronobiologia*, vol. 3, no. 1 (January–March 1976):75–76.

Halberg, J., E. Halberg, F. Halberg, Proceedings of the 10th International Congress on Nutrition, Kyoto, Japan, August 1975, Abstract No. 211, p. 16.

Hirsch, E., F. Halberg, F. C. Goetz, D. Cressey, H. Wendt, R. Sothern, E. Haus, P. Stoney, D. Minors, G. Rosen, B. Hill, M. Hilleren, K. Garett, "Body Weight Change During One Week on a Single Daily 2000-Calorie Meal Consumed as Breakfast or Dinner." *Chronobiologia*, supplement 1 (1975):31–32.

Jacobs, H., M. Thompson, E. Halberg, F. Halberg, R. C. Graeber, H. Levine, E. Haus, "Relative Body Weight Loss on Limited Free Choice Meal Consumed as Breakfast Rather Than Dinner." Paper delivered to 12th Annual Conference of the International Society for Chronobiology, August 10–13, 1975, NIH, Washington, D.C.; abstracted in *Chronobiologia*, supplement 2 (1975):33.

Chapter 8. Your Body Is Regulated Like a Clock

Aschoff, J., ed., *Circadian Clocks*. Amsterdam: North Holland Publishing Company, 1965, 479 pp.

Aschoff, J., "Circadian Rhythms in Man." *Science* 148 (1965): 1427–1432.

Aschoff, J., "Circadian Systems in Man and Their Implications." *Hospital Practice*, May 1976, pp. 51–57.

Chovnick, A., ed., *Biological Clocks*. Cold Spring Harbor Symposia on Quantitative Biology, vol. XXV. Cold Spring Harbor, N.Y.: The Biological Laboratory 1960, 524 pp.

Colquhoun, W. P., *Biological Rhythms and Human Performance*. New York: Academic Press, 1971, 283 pp.

Fox, C. A., A. A. A. Ismail, D. N. Love, K. E. Kirkham, J. A. Loraine, "Studies on the Relationship Between Plasma Testosterone Levels and Human Sexual Activity." *Journal of Endocrinology*, vol. 52, pp. 51–58.

Graeber, R. C., R. Gatty, F. Halberg, H. Levine, *Human Eating Behavior: Preferences, Consumption Patterns, and Biorhythms*. Natick, Massachusetts: U.S. Army Natick Research and Development Command, Technical Report, 1978.

Halberg, F., "Chronobiology." *Annual Review of Physiology* 31 (1969):675–725.

Halberg, F., E. Halberg, C. P. Barnum, J. J. Bittner, "Physio-

REFERENCES

logic 24-Hour Periodicity in Human Beings and Mice . . ." in *Photoperiodism and Related Phenomena in Plants and Animals.* Washington, D.C.: AAAS, 1959, pp. 803–878.

Halberg, F., E. A. Johnson, W. Nelson, W. Runge, R. Sothern, "Autorhythmometry: Procedures for Physiological Self-Measurements and Their Analysis." *The Physiology Teacher* 1 (January 1972):1–11.

Jenner, A., "Biological Rhythms and Human Behavior," in *Time: The Fourth Dimension of Medicine.* Symposium on the Clinical Implications of Chronobiology, New Orleans, November 3–4, 1973.

Kanabrocki, E. L., L. E. Scheving, F. Halberg, R. L. Brewer, T. J. Bird, *Circadian Variation in Presumably Healthy Young Soldiers.* Document PB 228427. National Technical Information Service, U.S. Department of Commerce, undated, 56 pp.

Kripke, D. F., "An Ultradian Biologic Rhythm Associated with Perceptual Deprivation and REM Sleep." *Psychosomatic Medicine* 34 (May 1972):221–234.

Lagoguey, M., F. Dray, J. M. Chauffournier, A. Reinberg, "Circadian and Circannual Rhythms of Urinary Testosterone . . . in Healthy Adult Men." *International Journal of Chronobiology* 1 (1973):91–93.

Lavie, P., and D. F. Kripke, "Ultradian Rhythms: The 90-Minute Clock Inside Us." *Psychology Today* 8 (April 1965):54–56.

Luce, G. G., *Body Time: Physiological Rhythms and Social Stress.* New York: Bantam, 1973, 411 pp.

Mills, J. N., "Human Circadian Rhythms." *Physiological Review,* vol. 146, no. 1 (1966):128–171.

Oswald, I., J. Merrington, H. Lewis, "Cyclic 'On Demand' Oral Intake by Adults." *Nature* 225 (March 1970):959–960.

Reinberg, A., and J. Ghata, *Les Rythmes biologiques,* 2ème ed. Paris: Presse Universitaire de France, 1964, 128 pp.

Richter, C. P., *Biological Clocks in Medicine and Psychiatry.* Springfield, Illinois: Charles C. Thomas, 1965.

Simpson, H. W., and J. G. Bohlen, "Latitude and the Human Circadian System," in J. N. Mills, ed., *Biological Aspects of Circadian Rhythms.* New York: Plenum, 1973, pp. 85–120.

Smolensky, M., F. Halberg, F. Sargent II, "Chronobiology of the Life Sequence," in S. Ito *et al., Advances in Climatic Physiology.* Tokyo: Igaku Shoin, 1972, pp. 281–318.

Taub, J. M., and A. J. Berger, "Diurnal Variations in Mood as Asserted by Self-Report and Verbal Content Analysis." *Journal of Psychiatric Research,* vol. 10, no. 2 (1974):83–88.

198

REFERENCES

Weitzman, E. D., "Biologic Rhythms and Hormone Secretion Patterns." *Hospital Practice* (August 1976) pp. 79–86.

Wilson, R. H. L., E. J. Newman, H. W. Newman, "Diurnal Variation in Rate of Alcohol Metabolism." *Journal of Applied Physiology* 8 (1956):556.

Zuckerman, M., "Physiological Measures of Sexual Arousal in the Human." *Psychological Bulletin*, vol. 75, no. 5 (May 1971):297–379.

Chapter 9. How Mealtimes Modify Your Body Clock

Apfelbaum, M., A. Reinberg, D. Lacatis, "Effects of Meal Timing on Circadian Rhythms in 9 Physiologic Variables of Young Healthy but Obese Women During a Caloric Restriction." 2nd International Congress on Energy Balance in Man, Lausanne, March 14–16, 1974.

Aschoff, J., F. Ceresa, F. Halberg, eds., "Chronobiological Aspects of Endocrinology." *Symposia Medica Hoechst* 9. Stuttgart: F. K. Schattauer Verlag, 1974, 463 pp.

Barnes, B. O., *Hypothyroidism: The Unsuspected Illness*. New York: Crowell, 1976, 308 pp.

Fuller, R., and E. Diller, "Diurnal Variation of Liver Glycogen and Plasma Free Fatty Acids in Rats Fed Ad Libitum on a Single Daily Meal." *Metabolism* 19 (1970):226–229.

Gatty, R., "Rhythms in Human Appetite for Sex and Food." Paper delivered to the Society of Mathematical Modellers, New York City, February 15, 1977, 17 pp.

Goetz, F., J. Bishop, F. Halberg, R. B. Sothern, R. Brunning, B. Senske, B. Greenberg, D. Minors, P. Stoney, I. D. Smith, G. D. Rosen, D. Cressey, E. Haus, M. Apfelbaum, "Timing of Single Daily Meal Influences Relations Among Human Circadian Rhythms in Urinary Cyclic AMP and Hemic Glucagon, Insulin and Iron." *Experientia* 32 (August 1976):1081–1084.

Greene, R., *Human Hormones*. London: Weidenfeld and Nicholson, 1970, 256 pp.

Jarrett, R. J., I. A. Baker, H. Keen, N. W. Oakley, "Diurnal Variation in Oral Glucose Tolerance." *British Medical Journal* 1 (1972): 199.

Jores, A., "Die 24-Stundenperioden des Menschen." *Med Klin* 1 (1934):468.

Kimura, T., T. Maji, K. Ashida, "Periodicity of Food Intake and Lipogenesis in Rats Subjected to Two Different Feeding Plans." *Journal of Nutrition* 100 (1970):691–697.

Levine, H., H. Jacobs, R. C. Graeber, M. Thompson, F. Halberg,

REFERENCES

"Timing Circadian Rhythm Characteristics for Physiologic, Physical, and Mental Performance of Subjects on a Limited Free-Choice Diet." Paper delivered to the 12th Annual Conference of the International Society for Chronobiology, August 10–13, 1975, NIH, Washington, D.C.; abstracted in *Chronobiologia* 1 (supplement, 1975):41.

Lakatua, D. J., E. Haus, E. M. Gold, F. Halberg, "Circadian Rhythms of ACTH and Growth Hormone in Human Blood," in L. E. Scheving, F. Halberg, J. E. Pauly, eds., *Chronobiology: Proceedings of the International Society for the Study of Biological Rhythms*, Little Rock, Arkansas, November 1971. Tokyo: Igaku Shoin, Ltd., 1974.

Nelson, W., F. Halberg, L. Scheving, "Meal Timing as an Adjutant of Experimental Chronotherapy." Paper delivered to the 11th International Cancer Conference, Florence, Italy, October 24, 1974; abstracted in *Chronobiologia*, vol. 1, no. 3 (July–September 1974): 315–316.

Nelson, W., L. E. Scheving, F. Halberg, "Circadian Rhythms in Mice Fed a Single Daily Meal at Different Stages of a Lighting Regimen." *Journal of Nutrition* 105 (1975):171–184.

Ostberg, O., "Circadian Rhythms of Food Intake and Oral Temperature in 'Morning' and 'Evening' Groups of Individuals." *Ergonomics*, vol. 16, no. 2 (1973):203–204.

Pike, R. L., and M. L. Brown, *Nutrition: An Integrated Approach.* New York: Wiley, 1975, 1082 pp.

Reinberg, A., "Chronobiology and Nutrition." *Chronobiologia*, vol. 1, no. 1 (January–March 1974):22–27.

Sargent, F., II, "Season and the Metabolism of Fat and Carbohydrate: A Study of Vestigial Physiology." *Meteorological Monographs* 2 (1954):68–80.

Sensi, S., "Some Aspects of Circadian Variations of Carbohydrate Metabolism and Related Hormones in Man." *Chronobiologia*, vol. 1, no. 4 (October–December 1974): 396–404.

Chapter 10. The Body Clock Diet

Bennet, J., and M. Simon, *The Prudent Diet.* New York: Bantam, 1973, 335 pp.

Jolliffe, N., *Reduce and Stay Reduced.* New York: Simon and Schuster, 1952, 235 pp.

Jolliffe, N., *Reduce and Stay Reduced on the Prudent Diet.* New York: Simon and Schuster, 1963.

Keys, A., "A Practical, Palatable and Prudent Way of Eating." *Journal of the Medical Association of Georgia*, September 1970, pp. 355–359.

REFERENCES

"The Prudent Diet." Bureau of Nutrition, Department of Health, the City of New York, revised 1974, 32 pp.

Chapter 11. Fiber Can Help Regulate Your Body

Burkitt, D. P., "Diverticular Disease of the Colon: A Deficiency Disease of Western Civilization." *British Medical Journal* 2 (1971): 450–454.

Burkitt, D. P., "Varicose Veins, Deep Vein Thrombosis, and Haemorrhoids." *British Medical Journal* 2 (1972):556–561.

Cleave, T. L., "Varicose Veins: Nature's Error or Man's?" *Lancet* 2 (1959):172–175.

Hegsted, D. M., Statement before the Senate Select Committee on Nutrition and Human Needs, January 14, 1977, in *Dietary Goals for the United States.* Washington, D.C.: U.S. Government Printing Office, 1977.

Painter, N. S., "Unprocessed Bran in Treatment of Diverticular Disease of the Colon." *British Medical Journal* 1 (1972):137–140.

Plumly, P. F., and B. Francis, "Dietary Management of Diverticular Disease." *Journal of the American Dietetic Association,* vol. 63, no. 5 (November 1973):527–530.

Spiller, G. A., and R. J. Amen, "Dietary Fiber in Human Nutrition." *Critical Reviews in Food Science and Nutrition* 7 (November 1975):39–70.

Spiller, G. A., and R. J. Amen, eds., *Fiber in Human Nutrition.* New York: Plenum, 1975, 278 pp.

Van Soest, P., "The Secret, My Friends, Is the Fiber." *Human Ecology Forum,* vol. 6, no. 4 (Spring 1976):1–4.

Chapter 12. Fiber Helps You Lose Weight, Too

Briones, E. R., P. J. Palumbo, R. A. Nelson, "Comparison of the Effectiveness of a Diet High in Unavailable Carbohydrate with Cholestyramine in Lowering Serum Lipids in Type IIa Hyperlipidemia." American Dietetic Association, San Antonio, October 23, 1975.

Colmey, J. C., and S. T. Titcomb, "Reduced Calorie, High-Fiber Bread, Energy Intake and Obesity." Workshop on Fiber and Obesity, Conference on the Role of Dietary Fiber in Health, sponsored by the National Institutes of Health, Bethesda, Maryland, March 28–30, 1977. Proceedings to be published.

Heaton, K. W., "Food Fibre as an Obstacle to Energy Intake." *Lancet* (December 22, 1973):1418–1421.

Kaunitz, H., Paper delivered to the 10th International Congress on Nutrition, Kyoto, Japan, August 3–9, 1975.

REFERENCES

Mickelsen, O., D. D. Makdani, R. H. Cotton, S. T. Titcomb, J. C. Colmey, R. Gatty, "Weight Loss with a Reduced-Calorie, High-Fiber Bread." Paper submitted for publication, December 1977.

Mickelsen, O., R. Gatty, D. D. Makdani, G. Williams, R. H. Cotton, J. C. Colmey, "Home Dieting with Reduced-Calorie, High-Fiber Bread and Behavior Modification." Paper submitted for publication, December 1977.

Stuart, R. B., and B. Davis, *Slim Chance in a Fat World: Behavioral Control of Obesity.* Champaign, Illinois: Research Press, 1972, 245 pp.

Stunkard, A. J., "From Explanation to Action in Psychosomatic Medicine: The Case of Obesity." *Psychosomatic Medicine,* vol. 37, no. 3 (May–June 1975):195–236.

Titcomb, S. T., "The Use of Reduced-Calorie, High-Fiber Bread in Special Diets and Weight Loss Experiments." Paper delivered to the 61st Annual Meeting of the American Association of Cereal Chemists, New Orleans, October 5–8, 1976. Reprinted in *Cereal Foods World,* Fall 1977.

Chapter 13. How to Change Your Eating Habits Permanently

Ferster, C. B., J. I. Nurnberger, E. B. Levitt, "The Control of Eating." *Journal of Mathematics* 1 (1962):87–109.

Stuart, R. B., "Behavioral Control of Overeating." *Behavioral Research* 5 (1967):357–365.

Stuart, R. B., and B. Davis, *Slim Chance in a Fat World: Behavioral Control of Obesity.* Champaign, Illinois: Research Press, 1972, 245 pp.

Stunkard, A. J., "From Explanation to Action in Psychosomatic Medicine: The Case of Obesity." *Psychosomatic Medicine,* vol. 37, no. 3 (May–June, 1975):195–236.

Chapter 14. The New You and How to Stay That Way

Bruch, H., *The Importance of Overweight.* New York: Norton, 1957.

Comfort, A., *The Joy of Sex.* New York: Simon and Schuster, 1972, 255 pp.

Nisbett, R. E., "Starvation and Behavior of the Obese," in G. A. Bray and J. E. Bethune, eds., *Treatment and Management of Obesity.* New York: Harper & Row, 1974, pp. 45–57.

INDEX

INDEX

protein-sparing fast, 44–47
Psychology Today, 48
pulmonary embolism, 156

Queen Elizabeth College, 29

Ramadan, 43
Rock Reproductive Clinic, 94

St. Luke's Hospital Center
  (New York City), 170
St. Paul-Ramsey Hospital, 75
Samoans, 28
Sassoon, Beverly and Vidal, 142
Science Digest, 21
Sebrell, Henry, 125
sensory threshold, 99
sex, interest in, 90–94
sexual libido, 54
Slimming Club, 29
slow-wave sleep, 57
Smith, Ian D., 115
Smithsonian Institution, 88
South Sea Islands, 28, 43, 60,
  144, 149, 156
Spiller, G. A., 152
Stanford Heart Disease
  Prevention Program, 56
Stunkard, Albert J., 182
Sums Test, 103–5

Tahitians, 28
task performance, 102–5
testosterone, 90
Thomas, Donald W., 48
thrombosis, 156
thyroid, 119–20
thyroid stimulating hormone, 120
thyroxine, 120
"tired blood," 118
Titcomb, Stanley T. 160, 165,
  170

tobacco, effects of, 57
TOPS, 187
triglycerides, 55, 56
Tufts University, 31, 125
tyrosine, 98

ultradian rhythms, 17
University College (London), 192
University of Arizona, 38
University of Chicago, 158
University of Massachusetts, 17
University of Michigan, 192
University of Minnesota, 68, 75,
  76, 115
University of Paris, 115
University of Pennsylvania, 182
University of Sydney, 115
University of Wisconsin, 54
U.S. Air Force Medical Corps, 51
U.S. Army Medical Research
  Institute (Frederick, Md.),
  98
U.S. Tactical Air Command, 21
urine flow, 94

Van Itallie, Theodore, 40, 170
Van Soest, Peter, 156
varicose veins, 157
vasopressin, 94

Wadsworth Veterans Administra-
  tion Hospital (Los Angeles,
  Calif.), 44
Walter Reed Medical Center, 13
Weight Watchers, 41, 187
Williams, Gordon, 168, 170
Wilmore, J. H., 38
Winnie Mae, 88
Wood, Peter D., 56
Workmen's Compensation Board
  of British Columbia, 21

Zen of running, 62

ABOUT THE AUTHOR

Dr. Ronald Gatty is Professor in the Graduate Division of Baruch College, City University of New York. A specialist in the scientific design of research experiments, he has been a member of several teams of medical and nutritional scientists studying body rhythms, weight control, and the importance of dietary fiber. He has served as consulting expert to the Food Sciences Laboratory, U.S. Government Pioneering Research Laboratories.

Dr. Gatty is a frequent speaker on the topic of body rhythms and has published many technical articles in professional and scientific journals. He is a member of the International Society for Chronobiology, the American Statistical Association, the American Psychological Association (Division for Consumer Research), and the Association for Consumer Research. He earned an M.Sc. and Ph.D. at Cornell University.

Originally from Australia, Dr. Gatty lives in New York City and spends his summers in the Fiji Islands, in the South Seas, which was his home before he came to the United States.